Everything but the medicine

I0884901

Everything but the medicine

A doctor's tale

Lucy O'Hagan

MASSEY UNIVERSITY PRESS

Contents

Mihimihi

Nō Aerani ōku tīpuna.
Ka tū ahau i raro i te maru o Tititea
i te tahataha o Mata-Au
i te tai o te roto o Hāwea.
Ko tēnei taku mihi ki ngā tangata whenua o
Te Waipounamu, me te motu o Aotearoa.
Ko Lucy O'Hagan tōku ingoa.
Nō reira tēnā koutou, tēnā koutou katoa.

My ancestors come from Ireland.
I stand in the shelter of Mount Aspiring
on the banks of the Clutha River
and on the shores of Lake Hāwea.
I acknowledge the tangata whenua of the
South Island and all of New Zealand.
My name is Lucy O'Hagan.
Welcome, to all of you.

Who is the doctor writing this book?

A doctor's tale

A long time ago a young maiden with hairy legs and a love of stories went where few women had gone before: medical school. She wanted to help people, but the hallowed halls were daunting. The portraits of the deans, austere men, stared down at her as if to say: 'You cannot be a doctor and a mother. Begone.'

Learning to help people seemed to be a brutal process and she wasn't so sure about the type of doctor they were turning her into, but in the back row she met a gentle young man with a brown ponytail who liked to protest outside Miss New Zealand contests and to go to men's groups to talk about feelings, and there beneath a slide showing the embryology of the gubernaculum testis Hunteri, they fell in love.

They learned to be doctors together, although it was a long time before either of them dressed like a doctor. They were later taught by a wise but humble physician who believed that being human was as important as being clever, and with their newfound skills they went to a small mountain town in the southern island, where they met another doctor, a woman with sturdy boots, who proclaimed in her loud American accent, 'I am strong, I am invincible, I am woman doctor. I am as good as those boy doctors. I will open my own medical centre.' She put up her sign and consulted patients in a sleepout behind an old cottage.

And the local people asked, 'Are you a real medical centre?'

And 'Does your doctor write prescriptions?'

And 'Can your doctor stitch up a cut knee?'

To their amazement she did it all, and before long there were queues of people outside the door.

Soon after, the young woman with hairy legs joined her, setting up her consulting room out the back door and down a path in the former garage, which had been given a flick of fresh paint, a new door and some easy-clean linoleum.

And soon the young man, who had grown into a gallant young doctor, joined the two women, and he did manly things like writing prescriptions and stitching up knees, but he also had a way with laughter that could ease the lowest of spirits, and he became famous for performing magic tricks for unwell kids.

Eventually they ran out of sheds, so they found a larger house with enough rooms for all their doctors and nurses. They were very prudent with money so they sewed their own curtains and made desks out of old doors held up with bits of four-by-two.

And they employed lovely receptionists, of all ages, who dressed more like doctors than they did, which was reassuring for the patients, and through thick and thin, day after chaotic day, those lovely receptionists sat at the desk made of a door, smiling and being welcoming and making appointments in a big green book using a pencil, with an eraser nearby in case there were cancellations.

And they also had nurses, who were not tea-making handmaidens; oh no, they were modern nurses, who had opinions and did pap smears, and managed the whole outfit, so that everything was ready and nothing had expired and things worked seamlessly.

Then they got managers, and the managers knew how to put numbers in a wide black book called *Cash Flow* with different-coloured ballpoint pens for different columns and white-out in case there were adjustments.

Later another doctor, a calm English woman, joined them and soon there were so many patients that brown folders of notes filled every corner of the large cottage and there was barely space in the staffroom to have a nice cup of tea.

They were young and modern, so they soon got a computer, and gradually all the green books and pencils and white-out and brown folders and self-carbonating pads and erasers were put in the shed out the back.

Some years later, the young man, who was now balding, proclaimed, 'We need more space. We must join the boy doctors and build a modern health hub.' And so they got together and built a type of 'med mall' where you could have a coffee and then browse the various services and decide whether today was for your teeth or your eyes or your shoulder or your blood pressure, or perhaps just a chance to buy a little tin of Vicks VapoRub.

In this modern health hub the desks were made properly by a man whose job it was to make desks and there was no sewing of curtains, just the endless writing of cheques. The people who used to write numbers in books now had a computer too, and their computer said, 'Yes, the books will balance', and they did.

+

By then the young woman had shaved her legs and the young man wore the occasional collared shirt. They had built a house in the countryside and had two boys, who therefore had the misfortune of having two parents who were doctors.

The young woman loved being a doctor. She loved stitching wounds and scary emergencies and demanding patients and sad patients, and she developed a curious concern for those with mysterious ailments that could not be categorised, and she found that sometimes it wasn't obvious what ailed people or what helped them. She came to realise that the gubernaculum testis Hunteri was seldom the problem, and a prescription was often not the answer.

She had a curious nature, so she asked questions, and the more she asked, the more she learned.

And the more she asked, the longer it took.

And the longer it took, the more the patients waited.

And the more they waited, the harder the receptionists smiled.

And still she sat in her room, asking and listening.

And she came to understand that she was hearing stories.

And as time went by, she began to see she had her own story.

Postscript: The gubernaculum testis Hunteri is an obscure piece of foetal anatomy that guides the testicle into the developing scrotum. Such information one learns and quickly forgets.

The case of Dr J. J.

Some time after my father died of a rare lymphoma, his lovely haematologist presented him as a case at a grand round. My memory, from my time as a medical student, is that a grand round involved a lecture theatre full of doctors and professors, mostly men, in white coats. A couple of the white coats would present the case of a patient who had some interesting diagnostic or treatment challenges.

Case reports in medicine are a very stylised version of events, always starting with 'Patient X was a X-year-old woman/man who presented with . . .' My father's case might have started with 'Dr J. J. was a sixty-nine-year-old man with a five-year history of benign chronic lymphocytic leukaemia (CLL), who presented with discomfort and distention in his left upper quadrant'. I imagine the haematologist would have described his symptoms, the physical examination findings and the results of his laboratory tests, perhaps showing slides of his biopsies, his cells with an unusual pattern for lymphoma, and she might have solved this diagnostic riddle by referring to a search of the medical literature, describing similar cases of this lymphoma, a rare complication of CLL.

The thing that is poignant about this story is that for many years my father, as the postgraduate dean, had chaired these grand rounds. He would introduce the speakers and at the end of the case presentation take questions and comments from the audience. Invariably the white coats in the audience were probing, and incisively competitive, and the presenter was always slightly on the back foot, needing to hold their end up, so the grand round was quite a tricky event to chair.

To help you understand the dynamic, let me describe my father. He had a good word to say about, and to, everyone. But he was deaf. He had one dead ear from a surgical misadventure in his thirties, which he never complained about. The other ear had survived surgery but needed a hearing aid. He made up for this disability with oodles of charm passed down from his Irish ancestors, so he had an uncanny ability to sail through the white coats, smiling and joking, often not hearing what was being said.

His mother was widowed early, and he was the first person in his family to attend university, but he had a strong sense of purpose. His favourite line was, 'Rules are made to be broken', meaning that the merits of every rule needed to be assessed and a decision made about whether that rule was worth obeying. He loved ideas, believed we could make things better, make a difference. He relished being challenged by his kids, as though the younger generation were pushing him to think harder and more creatively. He had three feminist daughters and two sons who learned early how to change nappies, so he had his work cut out holding his own end up.

To his credit he spent a lot of time thinking about women in medicine and the challenges to the old order. He famously invited Sandra Coney to speak to a grand round. She was the feminist journalist who had exposed the abusive and unethical research that led to the 1988 Cartwright Inquiry into Allegations Concerning the Treatment of Cervical Cancer at National Women's Hospital. Sandra Coney wasn't usually invited to speak to rooms of white coats but, as I have said, my father liked to break the rules.

Perhaps he is most remembered for his way with patients. He

was the only specialist who would sit with the patient during the ward round. Never mind the trail of junior doctors and medical students standing around the bed, he would find a chair and sit, his eyes level with the patient's, giving them his full attention.

+

And so, over those years that my father chaired the grand round it was convivial and energetic, and he always managed to steer the conversation to his own agenda, putting out his own challenges and wonderings. My enduring memory as a medical student is of watching him manage his deafness during question time. There was no such thing as a cordless roving microphone then, so it was pretty hard to hear the questions being asked. For the benefit of the audience my father would repeat the questions, or rather he would catch a few key words then turn it into a question that he thought was useful or interesting and then tell the contributor what an excellent question they had asked. He got away with it through sheer force of energy and enthusiasm.

A few years later, when the case of Dr J. J. was presented at the grand round, my mother was invited to attend and sat in the back row. It was very unusual for family members to ever be allowed to hear the discussion of a loved one's case. Occasionally patients might be wheeled in so the doctor could demonstrate a particular physical finding for the edification of the other white coats. But in my father's case, by the time he was presented he had died.

In telling this story, my mother described a rather dull, indecipherable presentation which ended with the haematologist putting up a photograph of my father. This was also unusual; case presentations did not involve identifying images of the patient being discussed.

But there he was, my father, larger than life, smiling down on the lecture theatre. It was now question time but for the first time ever, there were no questions. There was complete silence, my mother said: no raised hands, just an extended moment where the *case* in all its pruned medical austerity suddenly became a person, one they all knew and loved.

And after an awkward moment of hesitation, unexpectedly, they all clapped.

The inhabitants of the house with the turret window

I was brought up in a rowdy house in Invercargill with a turret window, warm kitchen and a coal shed out the back. The interior was full of older siblings who seemed to be perpetual teenagers, naughty teenagers, who wanted *peace*. My grandfather and his First World War cronies called them long-haired louts. The Marist brothers who taught them often sent them home to have their hair cut above the collar by my mother, who wore a pink kaftan and had a poster of Jimi Hendrix in the kitchen.

It was a home full of robust dinner table conversation, where the main topics were politics, sex and religion. Many years later I learned, by terrible faux pas, that in the best of circles politics, sex and religion should not be discussed at dinner, or at all.

We laughed with gusto. We showed affection by 'taking the piss' or what you might call 'making fun of each other', which I have also discovered is not a style found in polite society.

My mother taught me about words and the importance of being able to stand up and speak, whether it be a speech for a conference or a ditty for a birthday party. I can still feel her red pen hovering, about to correct my split infinitives, while telling me she loved it.

My brother Sean, the oldest, commandeered the storeroom beside the coal shed as his space. There he hosted gatherings of long-haired louts and girls who looked like Nana Mouskouri.

At 10, my sister Mary was taken to visit the priest because she had told the nuns she didn't believe in miracles. My mother was summoned, but I think perhaps the pink kaftan gave her away as the problem. My mother retold the story, both with and without shame, but in great humour as if to let us know that even high priests can be absurd.

Next was my older sister, Shonagh, who was my main playmate; dolls, knucklebones, last card, sewing. If we were hungry, we would cook pots of Edmonds custard or ransack the house for loose change to buy a packet of MallowPuffs at the dairy. If my mother knew we were going she might ask us to pick up a pack of Tiparillos, the thin cigars she favoured in an attempt to look elegant while smoking less. My father called them an oral contraceptive.

Trips to the dairy for Tiparillos were so regular that one day the shop girl asked, 'Again? Do you eat these things?'

Back then my mother would spend hours with Shonagh in the turret window, teaching her to read. She was severely dyslexic. My father lived by the maxim 'There is an opportunity in every threat', and Shonagh took this to heart, taking adversity in her stride.

The much younger one was Liam, full of giggles and bouncing curls. With three feminist sisters who all became working mothers, he was perhaps destined to become a stay-at-home dad, a role he took to with humour and purpose. And before Liam there was Dominic, who died when he was just five days old from a heart defect. We saw the small white coffin go into the ground and learned why adults sometimes cry.

I was the fourth child, and my siblings seemed to need my parents' help with life or reading or nappies, so I took to being self-sufficient. As one does in big families, I learned a lot about life from observing, and from being buffeted by the rowdy, good-natured chaos.

The holiday death toll

For as long as I can remember, the summer holiday period has been accompanied by the holiday road toll and, to a lesser extent, deaths by drowning or freak accident. You might wonder why these deaths are news at all; perhaps it serves as a coded warning to be careful, slow down, watch our step.

The holiday death toll is somewhat theoretical until one of the names released is your brother.

My brother Sean.

His life was a short sentence full of subclauses: he studied social anthropology, trapped possums and turned them into sausages, wrote the history of Otago rugby — a game he had never played — and married a Samoan woman, with whom he honeymooned in the rain up the Albert Burn as he researched the script for a documentary on the 45th parallel.

And then one day, aged 28, he was gone. Swept away down the Haast River, his body never found.

Recently I visited the bend in the river where Sean drowned. It is big country, granite peaks, dark bush and the sense of nature's life force, both beautiful and brutal. The rain was pouring down as it had been the day we searched for him, mist floating above trees, clouds of sandflies, the river, usually a charming trickle, now an ominous surge.

I had never visited the place in bad weather. We have always saved the pilgrimage for nice sunny days, not exactly having a picnic but at least feeling uplifted in the sense of being reminded, but with poignancy rather than devastation. But this time there was a grimness.

Standing in the rain I was taken back to another memory, of being the younger sibling, joining Sean on one of his solitary outings into the bush. I say solitary because we seldom spoke; we were both afflicted with our family's need to be in one's own head and we could handle companionable silence. He took me up a valley with no tracks, made mānuka tea in a billy over a fire, using water from the creek. We shared scroggin. I am weeping, now, remembering.

The sudden death of a young person is gut-wrenching, and Sean's death had a profound effect on my experience of living. If you have not had such a loss, you have been lucky. I was 21 and thought I knew a bit about life, but I had no idea you could feel an emotion so big, the size and weight like carrying a skyscraper on your shoulders. It was isolating, but I can still remember the small acts of kindness, the light touch of a hand on my back, those who were not frightened to see the enormity of it.

My visit in the rain was exactly 36 years after Sean had fallen while crossing the river. He was never seen again. Even after all that time I had a moment that day, which came out as a strange question to my partner: 'Do you think he did end up out to sea?' We had always imagined that the river had carried his body 47 kilometres down to the coast, and whenever I have visited South Westland I have imagined small atoms of him washing towards me in the surf, soothing me. But that day I had this terrible moment of thinking that perhaps all that time his body had been caught by an underwater branch then packed in with silt and maybe right now I was standing on his unmarked grave, not knowing. I felt sick.

It's the feeling that can come back, even now, decades later, out of the blue, a physicality, an embodied sensation of violent extraction as if suddenly losing part of oneself. The death of a child creates a big dark hole in a family. My mother says she lost a decade of her life grappling with filling it in.

If you have had a loss like this, I acknowledge the enormous load you carry. Our stories are all different, but I wonder what it is like to have a child die of a brain tumour, or a suicide in your family, or a parent drop dead in front of you.

This year over the summer I have noticed that, over and above the road toll, there have been almost daily reports of murder, and that gives me the same sick feeling. I wonder what it would be like to have my brother's life, or my child's life, taken by another and what sort of story I might be part of for that to happen, and I feel lucky. And I can't say why I feel lucky because I am weeping again. It will pass.

Caution. Patients.

I have a photo of my sister Mary, cut out of a newspaper. She is young, her gaze is a mix of innocence and 'don't mess with me'. She is standing in the driveway of a large psychiatric hospital. Behind her are huge rhododendrons and a sign. The sign reads, 'Caution. Patients.'

I am 17. I am visiting my sister, who is in a locked psychiatric ward. For some reason the keys are enormous. The smell is disinfectant mixed with ashtray. There is a sense of menace, as if something could suddenly happen, but I am unsure where the threat is located. My sister is in a room with a peephole and a grey blanket. She is so drugged, she drools. She is 23.

Years later we are driving in a car together. Mary is now an internationally renowned advocate for psychiatric survivors and a mental health commissioner. I am a doctor, a somewhat suspicious occupation from her viewpoint but, more importantly, we are sisters. There is a moment where she says, 'Peer support for people in mental distress is as good as anything doctors or psychiatry or therapy can do.' And even though it jarred me, I knew there was a truth in it.

I am a teenager, in my family home. I wake to an anguished cry. It's Mary. My mother goes to her. The lows have got so extreme that she cannot move or speak. After a few days she is back in elation, mania dancing her to the radio while the rest of us eat a sleepy breakfast. When the news comes on, she dances to that, too.

I have a video of Mary and her partner Sara and their three little kids, and Glen and Robert, the fathers of their boys. It is a TV documentary about queer families, and for some reason at the end they bring on a Catholic bishop to put in his 10 cents' worth. It's enraging. But Mary, in her forthright way, always with a chuckle, says something like, 'Well, I'm not sure a celibate man in his eighties who has never had a family has anything worthwhile to tell us about how to bring up kids.'

We are at the GP conference. I am watching my sister enter a panel discussion about mental distress. Her voice glides in, perfectly pitched to elicit some sort of humorous self-deprecation in the professional audience. As if it is obvious, she says something like, 'Of course, GPs can be specialists in earnest grandiosity.' I have to admit, I had a chuckle at my own grandiosity.

I'm holding a book called *Madness Made Me* by Mary O'Hagan. To my amazement a doctor beside me says, 'That book changed my life.'

Decades later, the sign is gone, but we are still grappling with the concept of 'patient' and what needs to replace 'caution'.

My mother is dying, and I am lucky

My mother is dying, and I am lucky.

She says she is lucky.

'I am at the end of a great life,' she smiles.

I am lucky she didn't die last year on that long night drive to hospital. None of us was ready.

I am lucky we can care for her at home. I'm lucky my family all get on, that we know how to laugh. And cry.

I am lucky to live in a country with a welfare state that pays for palliative care, commodes, catheters, medicines, carers and hospital beds.

I am lucky my mother is affluent enough to buy herself a wheelchair and a La-Z-Boy and lives in a home that is warm and roomy enough for grandkids on the floor.

I am lucky to be entitled enough to request more catheter bags or more care. That I can afford to take time off work to be with her.

I am lucky to work for people who understand whānau and what matters in the end.

My mother is dying, and I am lucky.

I am lucky to have a mother who has loved me, encouraged me, believed in me.

I am lucky to have had a mother who believed in herself.

I am lucky to have had a mother with the imagination to be

tolerant, who welcomed everyone into her home. The worst offence one could commit in my mother's world was to be *tricky*. That's as bad as a person can get.

I am lucky to have a mother who can recite verbatim Milton's 'On His Blindness' in ED with oxygen saturation levels less than 60. I am lucky the doctor tending her knew the sonnet and joined her for the last line: 'They also serve who only stand and wait.'

I am lucky to have a mother who wants my partner and ex-partner at her table, together, who accepts her children's unconventional paths, with gusto.

I'm lucky we have had this year. We have had fun. We had a farewell family party nine months ago. We all did items, as we do. Her own message was, 'What matters most is caring for people, treating others well.'

The next day we planned her funeral.

'My death is a sort of adventure,' she says. 'Or maybe just an event. But you have to stage an event properly.'

My mother is dying, and I am lucky.

I am lucky to see my mother naked. I am lucky I can wipe her bottom for her, that she can laugh when she finally opens her bowels, and we all clap.

I am lucky my partner will drop her life to come. A sister-in-law who will give Mum a hug at 4 a.m., after cleaning up a mess. Sisters who never doubt the value of caring.

And Grandma's vision of loveliness: my niece, so soft and calm. Her Samoan mother, my drowned brother's wife, who arrives always with flowers, gentleness and four cooked chickens. And a busy sister-in-law who encourages my youngest brother to travel halfway around the world, multiple times.

I am lucky to have a mother who smiles every time a grandchild enters her room, who posts randomly on the teenagers' Facebook pages, who is still curious about their worlds. I am lucky to have a mother who at 86 is a role model for her 19-year-old gay grandson.

I am lucky to have a mother who has taught me the language of life. And love.

My mother is dying.

And I am lucky.

Much luckier than some.

Death at home

My mother died at home, surrounded by family. We read her Lauris Edmond and Hone Tuwhare and she seemed soothed. Then she took off her oxygen tubing, removed her hearing aids, and demanded tea in a cup.

'I'm not having any more tea on one of those mouth sponges,' she said.

At the first sip of tea, she coughed and gasped and heaved. Desperate, she propelled herself off the bed, knocking the chair sideways. As she fell I managed to catch her flailing body, and as I held her she whispered, 'I'm done. Just lie me down flat in a comfy bed like you promised.'

The promise of comfort, the promise of palliative care. But death, like birth, is hard, dirty, messy. I felt bad about the evenings of agitation my mum had suffered. She hadn't been soothed by the morphine liquid, clonazepam drops and midazolam spray; she just got more disorientated, and I got more distressed.

Maybe death has to be this way, gruelling and unbearable, because at some point we have to let go. To know we are done.

We were lucky. We had had one meeting with a lovely palliative care physician, who had changed Mum's life by reassuring her about her death. Palliative care nurse specialists visited weekly; they were practical and kind and engaged. A district nurse visited daily to change syringe drivers and draw up extra doses of drugs for us to give her overnight.

But that night, at 11 p.m., when I lay my mother flat on the bed, there was no one.

I had the number for an on-call district nurse but when I had rung a few nights earlier she had taken 30 minutes to get back to me. She also didn't seem to know my mum or have easy access to her notes.

I had a cell phone number for a GP I had never spoken to, who was covering my mum's GP, who was away. It wasn't clear whether he had agreed to be called at nearly midnight.

I knew her lungs would start to fill with fluid when we laid her down flat. Things were happening fast. I didn't have time to think about who to ring or where their numbers were, and I couldn't manage their middle-of-the-night sensibilities.

+

I didn't want to be managing my own mother's death, waking my siblings, telling them to come, deciding when to give the doses of morphine and midazolam. We had been left with five syringes of each. I did not want to be the one explaining to my family what was happening, what might happen next, what the medications were for, what the grunting was, what the quietening of her breath meant, how we would know.

I did not want to be watching on as my siblings wept and laughed and sang, drinking whiskey and tea while I was thinking, looking for signs of agitation, recording the medications, speaking softly into my mother's ear, making sure everyone had a chance to hold her hand, supporting those who had never seen death, and holding her pulse through her last halting gasps of life, and finally, after a moment of silence, declaring her dead.

I did not want to be thinking about what we would do now, who to tell, how long to pause before laying out her body, turning off the heating, removing her catheter, making sure sharps were disposed of and planning when to ring people.

I wanted to be a daughter at the death of her mother. But I was a doctor at the death of her mother. Exhausted and harrowed though I was, I did it and I did it well.

And looking back, perhaps if an unknown professional had entered into that dimly lit family scene, it wouldn't have been right.

And maybe my mother could let go, let herself be lain flat, because I was there.

An amazing thing happens when a doctor turns and faces you

I witnessed an amazing thing recently while observing a first consultation between a neurologist and a young man with epilepsy. She faced him, giving her full attention, gathering his story, clarifying and carefully considering. I watched her artfully engage with him while simultaneously weighing up complex clinical considerations.

A quiet female medical student was also in the room watching this transaction. The young man put on a good show, as patients do for the doctor, as if saying, 'Even though my life is a mess, I can still muster something for this event, because it matters.'

His life was a mess in a way. He had been a highly articulate schoolboy debater, then a political student journalist, but he had developed epilepsy in his second year at university. Although it was not explicitly said, it was clear to the neurologist that he was good at taking his medication, looked after his sleep and had given up partying. Although his mind had clearly once been the mainstay of his identity, he was pragmatic about his new reality.

The medical student looked on intently as the young man described how he had been well controlled for two years, but last August his seizures had mysteriously returned. Initially there were seizures weekly but despite that he had managed to finish his law degree by Christmas. He had been on a sickness benefit since his graduation.

The neurologist praised him for keeping a seizure diary in an app on his phone. It was a minimalist visual record of the explosions in his head that leave his mind so shattered that he now often leaves sentences unfinished or is unable to retrieve the precise word to express the nuance of his opinion.

The medical student's brow crimped slightly when he explained, somewhat objectively, as if he was a doctor reporting on himself, that due to the medication's side effects he had gained 20 kilograms and developed a hand tremor.

The neurologist took in the said and the unsaid. You could feel her mind intent on the task of assessing, analysing and planning. It was when she said that things were maybe getting better as there had been a month between the last two seizures, and therefore maybe the best thing was to stay on the same drugs for a bit longer; it was in that moment I knew I was going to cry.

I am that 24-year-old's mum.

I'm not sure what I said but it was something like, 'It's so painful waiting.' It's been a very slow process as each seizure brings a slight increase in dose, first of the levetiracetam and then months later, when that didn't work, a new drug: valproate. He was now on the maximum dose of both, but there had been another seizure the day before. Before we knew it, 15 months had passed, months when he should have been launching into his life, full of energy and ideas and invincibility.

I did cry, and the neurologist turned and faced me, and I felt the medical student lean in, gently. People have asked me what the neurologist said but I truly have no idea. I'm not even sure she spoke. I recall she handed me some tissues. I do know that I had a complete sense of her kind, steady acknowledgement, her knowing exactly how long to let the tears roll, and then her instinctively knowing how and when to gently move me towards the next steps.

+

I recall feeling OK that I was crying, that tears needed to be shed in the telling of this story, and even though my son now had his arm around me, supporting me, it was somehow right to show that a case of a 24-year-old epileptic comes with its own pain.

I wanted the medical student to know it is complicated, that it is sad to see my son in this situation, but that at the same time I am so proud of him, so proud of him for getting up each morning, for walking towards the big questions of life: Who am I, what really matters to me, how can I make my life, as it is now, a good life?

And I wanted to tell them about the good things, how much it helps when a stranger enters the story and says, 'Yes, I'll give this young man a break. He can help me with writing or research, just two hours a day.' And I wanted to tell them about the flatmates who in their loving, accepting and laughing way have taught me something about the care of the collective, of whānau.

My oldest son and I walked out of the hospital, arms looped together, feeling lighter, knowing we had a plan, knowing someone had listened and lessened the weight of it. That's the way it should be when you leave the doctor; you want to feel a little lighter, more hopeful.

It is incredible what can happen when a doctor turns and faces you.

Matemate-ā-one

A few years before Covid, when I was still gallivanting around the world as if the meaning of life was to be found somewhere else, I wrote about the best part of travel, returning home.

> *Home.*
>
> *I love that moment navigating some vaguely hostile airport halfway around the globe when I get to my gate and see the koru. And I know at the plane door I will be greeted with a hearty 'Kia ora' by a bloke with enormous hands and a sense of fun.*
>
> *And after a nasty egg omelette I will arrive early over the craggy hills of my country on the fringes of the earth, safely do a dawn walk along a green line across an airport and smell damp earth.*
>
> *Home.*

+

I am with a group at a noho marae, meandering around whakapapa, colonisation, belonging and home. The other manuhiri with me are Pākehā, tauiwi immigrants and urban Māori impacted by migration from ancestral whenua. I am reminded that belonging involves longing. Longing for home, for land, for connection: matemate-ā-one.

It's the same feeling I had recently, flying along Kā Tiritiri o te Moana the Southern Alps towards Central Otago, where I lived for 20 years. I was coming home.

Our attachment to place can be primal.

Hāwea Flat is a small rural settlement with a school, a hall and a church. To get there you take a side road off the tourist trail. When I return on a hot afternoon, a broad winged kāhu is drifting on the thermals above the clothesline. At dusk the belly of Kahuitamariki Grandview Mountain glows. At night, the Milky Way drapes over us. It is so quiet. Home.

We are staying in the family home I built with the father of my kids. I lived here for so long I understand the choreography of the kitchen and can remember when the native garden outside was barren paddock grass. Next door is the house on the hill where I lived with my new partner. Both home.

We all take a trip up to Kidds Bush, travelling along the edge of Lake Hāwea. We pass the Neck; before the lake was raised in the 1960s it was known as Manuhaea lagoon, a kāinga mahinga kai or traditional food-gathering site. I only just learned this, even though I have driven this road many times: as a child on family holidays, with my own children, on the night my brother was drowned. I have biked this road, taken babies for walks in backpacks, piled kids into cars for camps. But now, to be back in the bush, the mountain beech red-laced with native mistletoe, the birdsong, and from that ridge above the bushline, looking back along the length of the lake. That blue. Home.

There is a sense of the land in me, as much as me in the land.

I am now living in the North Island, a great adventure, but I have this disconnected feeling; I am in a land that is not in me.

After our walk we swim in the mighty Mata-Au Clutha River, floating along in the chilling clarity of it.

Today we walked up the Matukituki valley, where my younger son is working on the Aspiring Hut renovation. I first went to this hut as a six-year-old in Bata Bullets that blistered my feet. My mother consoled me with Chesdale cheese triangles wrapped in foil and Sunshine rice risotto for dinner. Half a century later Tititea Mount Aspiring still towers over us.

An English friend once took a Sunday drive up the Matukituki Valley's long gravel road to the start of the Aspiring track. 'I can't believe you can drive fifty kilometres and end up nowhere,' he said. I guess it depends how you define somewhere.

Home is a kind of somewhere. A somewhere that we long for.

I am back at the noho marae wondering about pepeha, colonisation, migration, belonging and home.

Ko Tititea te maunga, ko Mata-Au te awa, ko Hāwea te roto.

1.
Patient

Patient. In a medical story a patient is a character who is sick or suffering and seeks help from health services, which are staffed by people specially trained in the diagnosis and treatment of diseases. Patient is a term used almost exclusively in situations where the sick person is attending a service that uses and privileges the biomedical scientific model in approaching the person's problem.

Silver beet

Sometimes I remember long-ago patients with a dream-like quality, as if they are hovering just beyond sight, murmuring. Like the man who lost it, literally everything. I don't even recall his name; maybe it was Frank. It feels bad to say it, but my heart sank just seeing his name in the book, knowing his stoop was waiting for me.

He was a regular attender, and I am a running-behind sort of doctor, so Frank got to spend time with my receptionist, chatting about the kids or petrol prices or when to plant the spuds and whether the washing would dry. He liked women so he always felt better by the time he got to my consulting room, which was a relief as I felt I had little to offer him. I had watched him uneasily for years as he lost his business, his family, his home and, finally, his sanity. In the end he was left with only his car, so he slept in it.

I think I have blanked out what happened next. I know it bothered me. The car was small, and he was a big man, but who was out there to help? The social services were busy assisting people without cars. I was his doctor; I could hardly invite him to stay on my floor or offer him the shirt off my back, and I felt I was doing my bit for him — after all, his appointments were frequent and onerous.

Soon he parked his car outside our medical centre and slept there. I arrived one morning to find he had planted silver beet along the edges of our sandpit. An elderly neighbour had lent him gardening tools, but she didn't invite him in, so he stayed where he was, in our parking lot. It was disconcerting, him being there.

+

Thank goodness he was clean, taking advantage of the garden sprinklers on timer. And he was a friendly fellow, Frank. We were in a nice part of town, so the other patients greeted him politely, but seemed unsure what to make of him; after all, silver beet was quite an unfashionable vegetable.

We never discussed the Frank situation in staff meetings. What was there to say? We could hardly ask him to leave, to park elsewhere. So we let him in to use the loo at his convenience. Despite the conveniences on offer, he still stooped.

Part of me didn't want to look. I was busy with other patients and my own concerns. I wanted to divert him onto the weather, too, but as happens with these stories, we have a moment where we are compelled to glance, and he knew that I had seen, and there was a long pause until I found the word 'Sorry'.

Sorry about his mother who had died when he was born.

About his father who had lived on, drunk.

About his boyhood full of violence and violation.

Sorry about the pain of his gout, and that there was little I could give him for it due to his allergies and dyspepsia.

And sorry about the bill. He was, after all, no longer a man of means. He said he was happy to pay. Things were looking up. I had come across him, at the end of a long day, bent over a small patch of dirt between the 'doctors only' car park and the fence that hid the crushed cartons, medicinal waste and empty oxygen cylinders.

He was planting a row of Brussels sprouts.

'Great autumn crop,' he said.

He handed me a bunch of silver beet.

Lying to get him out of the room

'I just need a *P* endorsement on my licence.'

'Sure, we can do that,' I say. The homemade tattoo on his wrist says *fuck off*.

'So, why do you need a passenger endorsement?'

'My mate's giving me a job driving disability vans for kids.'

'Great,' I say, taking in the tattered leather jacket, the jeans poised as if they might suddenly spring into action.

He hands me the driver's medical form, partially completed. He's well, with good vision and hearing, and no medical problems that will prevent his request.

'Have you ever had a drink-driving offence?'

'Twice. Off my record now. I don't drink.'

'Fantastic,' I say. 'How did you manage to stop drinking?'

'I smoke dope now. It chills me out.'

I listen to his heart.

Bom di, Bom di, Bom.

'Have you ever injected drugs?'

'Hell no, I wouldn't touch that stuff. I prefer meth and MDMA and benzos.'

The room suddenly seems small, like those disabled kids.

Bom di, Bom di, Bom goes my heart.

'If you couldn't drive shuttles, what other work could you do?'

We both know the answer to that question.

I stare at the form, looking for divine intervention.

The wrists have disappeared into the leather pockets.

'I'm worried there might be a problem,' I say, trying to convey 'benign' across the chasm dividing our realities.

'How come? There's nothing wrong with me.'

'It's the licensing authority.'

I'm about to say something not quite true.

'If you're going to drive passengers, they'll need a urine test clear of drugs.'

The jeans spring to upright, the hands leave the pockets, and for a split second he towers over me. *Bom di, Bom di, Bom.*

Fuck off, says the wrist.

Forget it then, says the mouth.

And in a moment, he is gone.

The power of swallowing

For years he has suffered. Nothing is wrong and nothing is right, and indeed what ails him is still a mystery despite my regular visits. He does not seem to get better, the man in his hut with no power, and one cold tap and a long-drop loo up a grass path that I have managed to avoid using despite him offering me the convenience of it many times.

He regularly requests me but does not want anything I suggest. All my tests, medications, specialist referrals and even acceptance and commitment therapy seem repugnant to him, so I only occasionally speak, usually a question, although sometimes I get away with a wondering.

I mostly just sit in his ancient armchair and listen to matters that seem unconnected. I've often wondered if I might be more helpful to him if I took my gloves and multipurpose cleaner and wiped down the inside of this tin long-drop shack to make it more appealing to the visitors who do not come these days, but might if they didn't have to face squatting above the dark cavernous collection of his shit and could relax on a clean seat.

And I get them, those visitors who don't come. It's hard to swallow tea from a cup that's been rinsed in a bucket of grey water.

Despite these strange, perplexing, going-nowhere visitations, where I too felt vaguely violated, I found myself growing to like him.

On one particular occasion, in which I was subjected to the usual rank and spittle and sour milk but during which we also managed to laugh together at the utter silliness of the world beyond, on that particular day that seemed no different to the others, just as I put the teacup to my mouth and swallowed, out of the blue, he wept.

I've always wondered if we could have got there a bit quicker.

Confirmation of the absence of life

I have sometimes wondered what other doctors do in a room with a dead body. It is not a ritual I was ever taught. Once as a medical student I went with an indifferent house surgeon down to the morgue in the dank basement of a hospital to view a body. But that was it.

Mostly now, the dead I see are in rest homes. People often die overnight so I go to certify the death in the morning, on my way to work. The body has been laid out, the family gone, the funeral director not yet arrived.

The room is always empty and cold and very still. That is the first sign. The lights are off, curtains shut. The person must be dead because there is an unmoving rose lying on their chest and the clean sheet over their body is undisturbed.

There may be a suitcase packed with the person's life. Sometimes there is a photograph left out or carnations given in the last days. But there's no sign of slippers or yesterday's paper or spectacles or crochet not finished or half-drunk tea; these are the things of life, tidied away.

I'm not sure one could pretend to be dead. Once the body cools and greyness seeps in, you can sense the spirit gone. Even so, I stand by the bed and put a hand on their wrist. There is a stillness to a body even if it is not yet stiff. You don't really have to examine it to know there is no breath or feel the pulse to know it is not there or listen to the heart to hear its silence. But I do these things anyway.

And often, now, it is someone I have known for many years, although it can be hard to tell in the dimness, their face gone blank. I might have a silent chat to them or say their name with an *Oh* before it. 'Oh Freda.' 'Oh Maggie.' 'Oh Bert.' And I might put a hand on their head and, not stroke it, no. One doesn't stroke the skin of the dead; that is for the dying. More a light touch.

And then there is a silence. I have done my job but it's hard to leave without lingering for a moment.

Before going back into the world of the living, I wash my hands.
This ritual is recorded. 'Death confirmed, absence of vital signs.'
It always feels as if something else is needed, so I write RIP.

Finding things under the skin

There is a tiny yin-yang tattoo on the arch of her foot. In front of that, a 5-millimetre-wide callous. Solid skin built up over eight weeks.

'How did the glass get in there?' I ask, as if somehow the mode of entry might give me a clue as to the exit strategy.

'It was a bit stupid. I was running in the dark in bare feet. I tried to get it out myself.'

Her toenails are aquamarine blue.

The X-ray report is vague as usual. 'Glass in sole of foot.' Yeah, thanks, the sole is a big place.

I press at it with my thumbnail.

'Does this hurt?'

'No.'

'No.'

'Not really.'

'No.'

'Ouch.'

'Sorry.'

Time for the local anaesthetic with adrenalin. 'This bit will hurt,' I say. 'It can be hard to find a piece of glass. Do you want to sit up and look, or lie back?'

I pick up the number 11 scalpel.

'It must be pretty sore to walk on. What work do you do?'

'Hospitality.'

The scalpel goes deeper.

'You'll feel a bit of pressure.'

Bloodless sliced edges of callous appear. No glass. The hole is too small.

'I'm studying at uni too.'

'What are you studying?'

There are fine linear scars on her left forearm.

'Law.'

'Good on you.'

I focus on gently lengthening the incision. I want a bloodless field, a clean cut. I'm hoping I'll be able to see the glass glint in the surgical light.

'So, what sort of hospitality?'

'Um. Escort.'

'How long have you been doing that?'

'A year.'

I pick up the fine mosquito forceps and stretch the wound, penetrating the subcutaneous tissue then stretching again. No glass. Bugger.

'How do you find it? The escort work, I mean?'

'It's OK, it's good money.'

I try the scalpel again. Sometimes fine layers of tissue can wrap around a foreign body. But I go gently, light pressure on the blade, hand steady. Then the forceps. Often you can't see the glass because it's gone deep, but you can feel it, almost a faint sound as the metal tool scrapes it.

'I've always wondered what it's like doing escort work.'

'You get used to it. Just switch yourself off, go through the motions.'

I breathe, relax my shoulders, move the probe into the depths of the wound, feeling my way gently.

'You must be pretty brave,' I say. 'There's some dodgy guys out there.'

Ting.

The hard feeling of metal on glass. The forceps go in, softly close, and out it comes.

'Yeah.

'That's how I cut my foot. I had to dump my heels and run.'

Visiting rites

a bath

the door was unsnibbed
I let myself in
she sat straight and still
I moved slowly across the carpet
close enough to whisper
asked what I had been taught

I wanted her to speak but she was silent
I said we needed to go
she nodded
I asked if she wanted anything
she said a bath

she did not move
we did not speak

I turned her taps
held her soap
washed her skin
towelled her toes
combed her hair
chose her clothes

then we went

no dog

tōtara crescent has a slow curve
the letterbox leans
the window is patched

hunkered on the carpet
near a strand of instant noodle
she stares at nothing

through her pregnant belly
I listen for a heartbeat

he is gone

but there is a sense of watching
distant children
yelling

and on the step
a dog's paw
rotting

but no dog

assessment with MallowPuff

I was asked to assess him
they were concerned

I bought a giant MallowPuff
and found him in a hollow
under his hedge
we drank tea in chipped cups

he talked of being watched
and followed
and taken away
by people wearing sunglasses
I had taken mine off

his veges grew in rows
he picked me some scarlet runners

I told them
he dreamed
of going to a quiet farm
with kind people
to rest

they said no such place existed

brothers

shingle road
macrocarpa
tin

I knock
the air inside stirs

in the dimness
white enamel mugs
on newspaper

a ninety-eight-year-old
is all I know

he is hollowed out
grey blanket
bare mattress
his woollen socks have a forlorn dignity

cautious
their eyes follow me

I try to be less
bright

there is a sense of resolution
a tenderness
as he caresses the hand
of the man
who is said to be
his brother

the ambulance waits
white
on the long grass
outside

on home visits

on home visits I have seen my consulting room
for the first time
how it is mine, not theirs
how they dress up to visit me
how formal and inhospitable we must seem
how much it resembles a stage
on which my visitors play the character
patient

Swallow that pill

Doctors are trained in a communication method called motivational interviewing, which can come out as a slightly patronising way of improving adherence or compliance so the patient takes the medications the doctor thinks are best.

However, as patients get older, they can develop multiple health problems that require different medications. Often patients in their eighties are still on the medications started in their sixties to stop them having strokes or heart attacks or kidney problems later on. This phenomenon of way too many pills is called polypharmacy.

Polypharmacy occurs in part because diligent doctors have, over many years, looked up their patients' ailments in evidence-based medical guidelines and prescribed the right thing for each different health condition.

The problem is that as people age they get more side effects, and some pills can interact with other pills, so things start to get complicated. GPs have the difficulty of deciding which medications to stop, and it's tricky because they have to balance the good evidence for why they prescribed them in the first place against the possibility of harm and sell any changes to the patient, who may well be attached to the pill they have taken for 10 years in the belief it was doing them good.

It all requires quite a lot of trust in the doctor's judgement, but even then, the patient still has to take the pills home and swallow them and, let's face it, swallowing small white chemically powdery things is pretty weird.

For example, it might be hard to warm to a pill with instructions like, 'Take before breakfast and remain in the standing position for thirty minutes.' It could feel like swallowing your school head mistress.

Doctors seem to assume pill taking is a neutral act done by a rational, health-literate patient who understands the evidence and robotically swallows as directed. But patients have their own ideas.

+

It's on home visits that I truly witness the idiosyncrasies of the pill–patient relationship.

'Those ones in blue foil are tough stuff,' he tells me. 'Sometimes I just don't feel up to taking them, so I don't.'

That's the dabigatran. I agree; the packaging makes them look radioactive and the fact you can't put them in a container with other pills is fairly concerning.

'But that one there, don't you take those away, that's my comfort pill.'

That's the omeprazole, for heartburn.

There's a giant Tupperware container filled up with tubes of urea cream, hydrocortisone, Soov, Chlorsig and Efudix alongside an ancient tin of Rawleigh's. He relates an elaborate system of when and where to apply them, not at all based on the instructions, which have worn off in any case.

He grabs the rolled-up end of a tube of Dermol and says he's saving that one because he knows I won't give him more, even though it fixes everything. Dermol is the strongest steroid cream there is and recommended only sparingly in the medical guidelines.

He has pills in bottles all over the place: on the top of the fridge, on a shelf in the shed, in the bathroom cupboard and on the bedside dresser.

In the laundry there is a box of about 700 paracetamol, from five years ago.

'I'm saving them too,' he says. 'They are the older brand that are easier to swallow.'

'What do you use them for?' I ask.

'I take them if I'm having a bad day.'

Beside his bed there is a small china egg cup containing two pills and two capsules.

'They are my wake-up ones,' he says. 'Before breakfast.'

'And where are your night ones?' I ask. I am relieved to see a plastic pack with a wee compartment for each day of the week.

'Very organised,' I say. But when I open them, Monday has thyroxine, Tuesday omeprazole, Wednesday zopiclone, Thursday and Friday Laxsol. Saturday and Sunday hold unidentified pills.

'What are these ones?' I ask.

'I think they are spares,' he says. 'I like a few spares.'

After a lengthy negotiation he consents to blister packs arranged in days and times by the pharmacy, but I can see they're not really wanted because somehow these pills are a man's final domain, like his shed.

The blister packs get sent back to the pharmacy. 'I'm not taking pills like that, they look like confetti. I've got my own system and it works.'

When do I admit defeat?

+

To be fair, it's good to have a system to remember pills. I'm the sort of person who would take contraceptive pills randomly on the wrong day of the week and I'm such a dreamer I can't remember if I actually swallowed a pill five minutes ago or just planned to but didn't.

It's easy to remember something that makes you feel better. But if a pill doesn't make you feel any different, what would make you swallow it? I'd have to trust my doctor and be scared of the consequences of not taking it, but then I would need some ritual around the moment of swallowing.

I have patients who say karakia before taking their pills and a prayer makes sense.

My mother quite literally called her pills her friends. 'I put them in my hand in the morning, look at them and say, "Thank you, my lovely friends, for keeping me going",' she said. 'Then I swallow them down.'

A bedsit

I remember her as naked
maybe an undergarment
purple lividity
where her hip had pressed the lino
that encircled the toilet
where her body lay

she had cut her head open on the way down

I do not remember her name
or why she had no next of kin

I had seen her before
for what ailment I do not recall
perhaps some troubles

what I remember is the glaring knowing
that some of us will die alone
and the feeling that the sun blazed too brightly
as I stepped outside

Explaining the legal limits to court shoes

'Well, Doctor, I use my car to visit my accountant, my lawyer, my stockbroker and my dentist. I do my shopping. What do you use your car for?'

Her court shoes gleam up at me.

'I mostly carry screaming children in mine.'

I instantly regret the *screaming*.

A driver's medical form appears between us. Her handbag clips shut.

'You will need to do an on-road driving test.' I stake a claim.

A single powdery cheek flickers. 'I knew your parents. He was very good.' My father was the Catholic doctor.

'Thank you. And congratulations on your hundredth birthday. That's quite an achievement.'

She had had a visit from the deputy prime minister. He is Catholic too. But blue.

I'm pretty sure she knows I am a bit pink.

'So, normally at your age we recommend you just use your car for local travel around the village.'

'And how, Doctor, will I visit my sister in Palmerston with that sort of restriction?'

I know there is no bus service. It's two mountain ranges away.

'Have you ever had an accident, Doctor?' she continues. 'I have never had one. In eighty years of driving.'

I feel myself relenting, then gird myself.

'And usually we recommend you only drive in daylight hours. Your night vision deteriorates as you age.'

'I have to disagree with you, Doctor. My eyes are excellent. And I prefer driving at night when the other cars have their lights on, because I can see them coming towards me.'

I look at the floor. The court shoes are tenderly tucked together in the shadow of her overcoat.

An aggro address

Nowadays I work at a free GP clinic in a dreary part of town between the prostitutes' collective and an ancient barber's shop. My room has no windows. It is so small there is no semblance of the appropriate distance between doctor and patient. I can see the sleep in their eyes. They can watch me blink.

There is no money for a computer because this is not a place attractive to philanthropists, or taxpayers, which is just as well because we could not fit a desk between us and still breathe. There is a landline, and outside the staff are ready for trouble. But inside there is just me and them, quietly absorbing the grime of life, redefining clean. The stethoscope is seldom necessary.

Today I met a beautiful man just out of prison. He's 28 tomorrow and trying not to drink. He has kids he cannot see because of protection orders. He told me he was raped at 10 and sentenced three times before he was 17, but it could have been worse. It could have been worse without his mum, who never gave up on him. But she's dead. And his sisters are all alcoholics.

I asked him what makes him feel good.

After a long pause he says, 'I like helping other people. But not the ones in gangs. I've done well to steer clear of them.'

'Yes, you've done really well.'

'That's what my aunty says. She's letting me stay in her garage.'

His aunty works in a factory that is closing down. For his birthday, I give him the form for the sickness benefit.

The next man, polite and shy, is carrying his possessions in a pillowcase. I know he has been couch surfing since his release but he has some pride, so he tells me he is staying with friends, only they are all alcoholics, which isn't good because he is trying not to drink. The address we put on the benefit form is the most stable address, but he doesn't want to live there because they're aggro.

I said he really deserved a home.

'No. Not really.'

'Yes, really, you deserve a place to call home.'

He took the form with the aggro address, stuffed it in the pillowcase and sloped away.

+

Today I have met men for whom prison is the nearest thing to home they know. Men who have never been safe, always vigilant. 'At least in prison people can't do really random stuff, there are guards. But you can't trust anyone on the outside.'

There is no safety except to hide, be on the run, punch the air in case it's mean. And I wonder, what is home if you have never had one? Do they have a tiny home inside them, these men, under layers of tattooed skin, below the sinew, inside the gut, hidden deep? A tiny home constructed from fragmentary moments of safety in a lifetime of crime; crimes inflicted *on* them, then *by* them. Do they carry this tiny home inside them when they run from the cops, rape their girlfriends and burgle our world?

So sometimes I ask, 'In your life has there ever been somewhere, or maybe someone, that felt good or safe?' And there is always something. Always a memory, a brief show of kindness, an uncle long gone, a mate who knew.

So yes, home can be carried, inside, and when it is seen, the light goes on.

Laying out

I'm not sure where I first heard the words 'laying out'. Perhaps in my childhood. My mother spoke of deaths, certainly drownings, in the village of Taieri Mouth where she had grown up, and maybe her mother was one of the women who went to help. It could have been a book or a film, set in Ireland, of course: a white sod cottage in a sea of green, women inside tending to the body, men out the back, drinking.

I had three older siblings so perhaps it was them, in their cheeky, breathless way, who told me you had to lie the body flat before it goes stiff ''cos if the knees are bent, they won't fit in the coffin'. They probably told me dead bodies can do poos and when you move them they can breathe out as if they are still alive.

At medical school rigor mortis and post-mortem lividity were forensic issues. Nurses dealt with the dead, behind closed doors. When I was a medical student, a nurse once showed me how to get the teeth back in and stop the jaw from sagging, but it was much later that I learned about turning the heating down. The room needed to be cool if there was a delay in the paperwork; usually the undertaker waiting for the doctor.

+

Long before that, in my first year as a GP, when I knew everything and nothing, I was called at night to a house where an elderly man had died. An expected death. A simple home with rhubarb at the back and roses at the front. And inside, his wife of 60 years. She must have done something to the lighting because the bedroom had a warm glow. I heard the story of her waking to a sound, and in a few minutes he had gone.

'Yes, he is gone,' I said.

She told me he was a good man. They had no children, no one who needed to be rung in the night.

I don't know if she had ever laid out a body, and my own knowledge was patchy. And I was a stranger in her home. But it seemed wrong to leave, so I suggested we wash him.

We got warm water and a flannel, starting with his face and ears, his head and neck, and then his chest and belly, thighs and feet, and finally a log roll so she could wash and dry his back. We folded an ancient towel and put it under his buttocks. Another under his chin. I don't think a word was said, although it must have been. Perhaps she whispered to him.

It's quite hard getting cotton pyjamas off a body in a dignified way in a double bed with an 82-year-old as your assistant. The dead are heavy. I was never taught to do this, but I was taught to look as if I know what I am doing. I may have wondered a few things like, what happens next, should I call the doctor (oh, that's right, I am the doctor) or do I call a funeral director in the night?

Or could she just get back into bed with him?

Maybe by then there was a neighbour making tea and maybe when we were gone the wife wondered if she ought to get into a twin bed in the spare room with cold sheets and pink candlewick and the smell of mothballs.

But no, I think she did go back and lie with him.

She told me they had never slept apart.

Board games

She smelt of death. But did not die.

We had done all we could, but her pain screamed on.

It was unbearable, to visit her.

On that day, her husband and small children stayed in the kitchen playing board games.

I made myself stay with her a while, but I don't want to sound heroic. I was consumed by my empty-handedness and fixed my gaze on a small sequence of stitching. Her bedspread was a soft pink.

Time passed.

I made myself still.

Not a word was spoken.

A fly landed, a distant child giggled, a truck went by, I steadied my breath, and not long after, she wept.

She wept as if her life depended on it.

I'd like to say that she took my hand but maybe that is not quite how it happened.

Time passed.

I made myself still.

Not a word was spoken.

A fly landed, a distant child giggled, a truck went by, I steadied my breath, and not long after, she died.

Lost prescription

A patient has requested her prescription early. I have never met her and there are no spare appointments, so I have agreed to ring her. Six weeks ago, she got another early script because she had dropped her pills into a waterfall. All of them: the morphine and diazepam for her, and the Ritalin for her son.

The receptionist tells me her regular doctor hadn't fallen for the waterfall story and had refused to give her a replacement script, but she had come in and yelled over the desk, only to be told it was now his afternoon off. So she had sat in the waiting room, under the 'Caring for you' poster, looking hard and limp, until the last doctor standing, a young GP, handed over the script, possibly so she could get out the door to her car without intimidation.

I rather like the waterfall story. I imagine the soggy trio of pills dissolving in the foam and floating away. Where would the waterfall be, I wonder? We are in the middle of an urban sprawl, and I am reading the notes of a woman on a sickness benefit with no car. So the rational bad cop in me is going, oh yeah, that's right, there is no waterfall. We're talking about the metaphorical river of diversion, the fact that most injected drugs are sourced from doctors who believe their prescriptions are for the patient's pain of life, but in reality the pills will be sold on to drug dealers and, sadly, other patients. I'm ready to pick up the phone and ring this woman with a righteous strut, knowing the generals from the war on drugs are at my back.

But then the good cop in my head says, well, she probably needs that money to feed her kids and how am I to know whether she takes it herself, or peddles it, or gives it to her son, or gets hassled to sell it? I could do a test to see if she had any morphine or diazepam in her bloodstream, but these people are not stupid; she could easily take the drugs before the test, so it looks like she is taking the pills.

In her notes I see a letter from three weeks earlier. She went to an after-hours doctor for an extra prescription, claiming the drugs had been stolen out of her car while she was at the beach with the kids. Beaches are a little closer to us than waterfalls, I guess, so the older GP relented. She got a week's worth.

I am putting off ringing her. Part of me is hoping she doesn't pick up, but of course she does, and she tells me the drugs were stolen off the kitchen table last night by some of her boyfriend's dodgy associates, who won't ever be allowed back after doing that.

And I'm back to bad cop, feeling emboldened because she is not in my physical space, and I'll probably never meet her.

I say, 'Well, you can't leave meds like that on the table, you have to lock them up, no one should know you are taking them and if your boyfriend has dodgy mates, then don't tell him where you hide them.

'You don't want to be put under pressure,' I say wisely, as though I know all about living in a house with trauma and drug-crazed violence and an empty fridge. But really, I'm saying, 'You need to do better than that, young lady, and I am going to consult my team, but I doubt we can give you an extra script', and I'm liking the idea I can say, 'No', mainly because there is now security at the front door, so she can't just walk in and yell over the desk.

'I'll get back to you,' I say, feeling the tide has turned. I will not be duped like that young GP or that after-hours doc. I am in control of this situation, and I will not be taken for a ride by her lies and deceit.

A second before I hang up the boyfriend appears down the phone, and I realise he has probably been there in the background all along, and I can feel a sweet, sinister, creepy sneer from him, and now I feel a bit weak, but I hold my ground.

I end the call and see five or six other patients who want normal things like Ventolin and blood pressure pills and reassurance, and I feel a bit better. But I know I have to ring her back and my clinical director has said, 'No, don't give it to her', but he has now gone home because he is more efficient than me, and I start hesitating.

My good cop starts thinking about the remote possibility she is taking the medications for good reason and has run out, and what if I don't give it to her and she goes into withdrawal — that would be bad — or what if she is in danger from that creepy boyfriend and will be beaten if she can't produce the drugs for him to sell.

I'm feeling weary and cornered again. So I work out the minimum I can give her for the next five days, just to prevent possible withdrawal, and I ring her back and say I will give her that much, and I get in my car and drive home and open my fridge.

+

Three days later, I will get a letter from the hospital. She will have been admitted with a smashed-up face, claiming she had fallen down a mountainside, and the doctors will have administered the equivalent of the 100 milligrams of morphine they can see she is regularly prescribed. She will have had a respiratory arrest, literally stopping breathing in front of her kids, who are sitting by her hospital bed, because, of course, she had never actually taken 100 milligrams and was well overdosed. The hospital will have brought her back to life and blacklisted her and refused to give her another script, but by the time her local pharmacy is informed the boyfriend will have already picked up the last repeat of morphine and likely sold it on the street, and the kids will have been put into the care of the boyfriend's uncle and aunt who, I will learn much later, have their own sinister way of bringing up kids.

And when all that unfolds and more, I will go home to a full fridge and wonder what story might have led her to this life.

I will make a donation to the food bank and feel a bit better. And then I will make another to the women's refuge so I can relax and enjoy deciding whether my next weekend away will be at a river, or at a beach, or in the mountains.

Face to face with suicide statistics

It was poignant, those 606 pairs of shoes on the steps of Parliament. Empty shoes, representing the 606 New Zealanders who had died from suicide in the past year.

Last week the son of my friend's brother took his own life. Tomorrow it might be a neighbour or a colleague. I think of my own children. Precious. I recently met a young woman who had been to eight funerals of young people who had died by suicide. She was 19.

Their spirits, known and unknown, hang on the horizon. They don't come back. We know the staggering grief of families, the wail of mothers. It's gut-wrenching, like just before throwing up; hollowing, like the moment after being punched. Is it the random unexpectedness of it? The finality? Is it imagining the body, grey and lifeless? Is it thinking of the person deciding to do it, alone, without worth or hope?

Some say suicide is a legitimate response to unfathomable suffering. But for the living, suicide is a terrible outcome. We know people can come back from that place, somehow the moment can pass. If there is that chance, what can we do to help as neighbours, friends, aunties, mates and health professionals?

GPs want to help people, so suicide risk makes us nervous. We openly bring it up. We have been taught how to assess risk, to ask if suicide is an option, whether they have a plan, and if they have the equipment. And we hope the answer is no because if it is yes, we get frightened. Frightened, because we know if we call the mental health team they may not come today because they are too busy, the situation is not bad enough, they are choking under the pressure of people with real problems.

And then we are left alone with the patient, our waiting room full. And what if we let them go home and what if they die?

+

I have been in this situation quite a few times. And I know that while I am racing through my suicide checklist and frantically phoning for help, something happens.

I turn away.

I leave the room.

I interact with the computer.

I have to make myself put the phone down, breathe out slowly, and look at them.

What story brought you to this place? What helped before? What has given you the will to live? Who loves you?

If I can stay steady then whoever they are, stranger or known, friend or foe, clean or unclean, I can find the love. There is always something beautiful. Something singular and strong.

Often I ask myself, 'If this person dies tonight or tomorrow or next year, what would I have wanted to have said to them right now?'

I usually say how devastated I would be if they killed themselves. I say this because it is true. I say there is always a way through, there is always hope, anguish passes. I say this because I know it is true.

I don't know if it helps. Maybe it just makes me feel better.

It's hard to stay steady when the stakes are high but I'm seeking the survivor in them, the bit that brought them in the door, trying to see the pieces of them they cannot see. And sometimes, something stirs.

I witnessed a miracle when we provided 24-hour care at home for a suicidal friend for a week. It was a labour of love. It worked.

I didn't learn this at medical school. I learned this from being alone in that room with the patient. Knowing I was not in control of whether they suicided. I was only in control of what I did in the next few minutes.

And yes, sometimes they die. And it is so traumatic. Death is final. We battle with ourselves. Did I do everything I could? Did I say everything I needed to say? How can I uphold this person's mana in the face of their decision? How do we support those left living?

Auē, auē, auē.

May that perpetual light shine upon them.

Cutting speaks for itself

After 15 years as a GP, I had had some profound experiences. I thought I was a pretty good doctor, in the sense of being able to respond to most of the challenges presented to me. Around that time, I was asked to join a theatre group that wanted to create a play about self-mutilation. I had done a lot of acting and I thought, rather grandly, that I was up to the challenge of inhabiting the experience of self-injury. So of course I said yes, and joined the Silk Tent Theatre Company.

We received a grant from the Mental Health Foundation and spent a year creating a multimedia theatre piece. I played the part of a woman who had experienced childhood sexual abuse and had cut herself repeatedly over many years. We were a community theatre group in a small town, but we took *Girl with No Words: Listening to the language of cutting* to audiences around the country.

I was the only health professional in the Silk Tent, but I soon realised I didn't have a monopoly on wisdom because of my medical degree. In many ways I had the most to learn. To create and act this character I had to stand in her shoes, respond as she would, hear her internal voices, be in her physiology, inhabit voicelessness.

This play changed me. There were huge shifts in my thinking about doctors and how we respond to distress.

+

Our research for the play was not like medical research, in which a problem is analysed through a detached academic lens, using statistical evidence. We wanted to hear real stories of self-harm and many people came to tell us about their experiences. Such individual stories are not valued in medical science; they are considered unreliable data, disregarded as anecdotal and too subjective. I had to dismantle this professional thinking and learn to listen differently, not with a doctor's ear, diagnosing and fixing, but instead letting something wash into my being so I could stand on that stage, and hold the blade myself.

People thought it was cool that I was involved in devising theatre. That was until the moment I told them the play was about self-mutilation. 'Or cutting,' I would add, feeling them recoil, repelled by the very idea of pressing a blade through your own skin. These were good people, their reaction was unconsciously embodied, not spoken. I saw how subtly our judgements can be communicated.

As a group, we pondered what is encased in this moment of recoil and wondered what compassion might look like. We talked about the power of small acts of kindness.

We realised there are cultural rules about expressing emotions. In our world a bloody self-inflicted wound is not on the list of appropriate ways to communicate distress. Crying is much more likely to elicit kindness than anger, or starving oneself, or swallowing razor blades, or impolite demands, or not turning up for appointments. But these behaviours can also be ways of communicating suffering.

I had doctored with the expectation that patients should talk to me in words, but I learned that many things are communicated only in actions, or by signals from the body. I came to understand that cutting speaks for itself. It is a language of injury on the skin, a way of managing the unmanageable. I gradually began to understand the interior world of self-harm and my own response to it. Why it helps. I ceased to judge it and I quickly realised that, as a doctor, *not judging* is one of the most powerful things I can do.

Sexual abuse was also not part of my experience but is a common story in people who self-harm for long periods. I read everything I could on the effect of trauma on children and adults and learned many things that were never taught in psychiatry.

I came to understand that abused children, if they survive, grow into adults, and those adults come into our medical centres with all sorts of problems that aren't easily explained: chronic pain, perplexing physical symptoms, anxiety, autoimmune disorders, relationships in which they are either abusers or abused, addictions, anger, tears and mystifying silence.

We tend to have much more sympathy for the traumatised children than for the adults they become. Adult trauma survivors are often labelled 'difficult' by health services. But their behaviours do make sense when we understand the drive abuse survivors have to keep themselves safe. Safety might mean throwing out anger, or being small and quiet, or not coming to a health service at all. I have taught myself to respond as if to the violated child within, giving that inner child kindness, telling them they will be OK. They are OK.

There is no psychiatric diagnosis that readily fits the experience of adult trauma survivors. Post-traumatic stress disorder (PTSD) covers some of it, but people who have been abused as children often attract diagnoses such as borderline or antisocial personality disorder. It's hard to imagine a label like that is good for anyone's self-esteem. What if, instead, we imagined them on a hero's journey? Then we might be prepared to sit with them, calmly, facing the horror of it, and seeing the strength it takes to fight the minotaur. Perhaps we could hand them a bundle of hope for the path ahead.

+

We spoke to many survivors of childhood violation, including a lovely young woman who had endured repeated rape and torture within her own family. Her story was hard to hear, viscerally sickening, and so horrific I marvelled at her continued existence.

She could barely tell us what had happened without going back into the trauma, convinced that we would abandon, punish or judge her.

Although I felt her wavering and her shame, I also saw her solid core of survivor. I learned that everything about her made sense when I understood her story. In that self-blaming logic of this abused child, she believed *she* must have been bad to have been treated so badly. She feared being observed, as though we might see through her, into her bad.

She contemplated death on a daily basis because she believed the world would be better off without a person like her. Her violated child was still carrying someone else's shame. She felt worthless, undeserving, at fault, faulty. She was constantly jumpy and on edge, as if something terrible was about to happen, because that was her experience. Horrific things did happen. But she had a grace about her.

As a child, she had learned to survive violation by disconnecting from her body, taking her mind somewhere else where she didn't feel the horror of it. Still now, at 33, she could suddenly dissociate from her body at any sign of threat. In that state, she was powerless over what others did to her, unable to speak, stuck in the physiology of trauma, until she got relief by cutting herself, feeling, and coming back.

She had learned how to tend her own wounds. When she cut herself, she never sought medical care.

She had been silenced by her abusers, threatened if she spoke and not believed if she did speak, so her tortured body carried an invisible story. She survived in a society where the rest of us don't want to know, can't believe these things happen, especially when the people claiming these abuses are beneficiaries, addicts, psychiatric patients, prisoners or 'borderlines'.

She said one day she hoped to tattoo her scars in gold.

She had recently been diagnosed with borderline personality disorder. She felt it was a terrible name, but she wanted a diagnosis because then she could get some help. But there didn't seem to be any help for people like her.

In *Girl with No Words* we considered the value of diagnosis. Does a label help? Or does a label start to define someone and limit their possible futures?

We discussed the whole ethos of recovery as a destination. Who defines that place of recovery, who says where it is and how to get there? And how might it feel to believe you will never get there, will always fail?

We talked of love. Loving the damaged child. Loving the one who seems difficult. Loving those who believe themselves unlovable.

This young woman had been through a labyrinth of terror and found unlikely mentors. She had learned who to trust, and what path was safe, by listening to her body.

She taught me how survivors of childhood abuse are constantly re-traumatised in situations where others have power over them. How as doctors, psychiatrists, police, judges and researchers we can easily and unconsciously become like the monsters blocking the path out of the labyrinth.

In *Girl with No Words*, I learned a lot about how we health professionals look through a patient's eyes. How in our well-meaning paternalism delivered in the structures of power we can do more harm than good. It is as if we have forgotten who the hero of the story really is.

+

A few weeks before opening night I read the then current Australian and New Zealand College of Psychiatrists' clinical guidelines on self-harm. I thought I should understand a medical view and the current 'evidence'. This document was far more disturbing than any of the graphic accounts of cutting I had read. It was a document of unexamined certainty, completely devoid of humanity or kindness. A document about self-harm in which the voices of those who self-harm were completely absent. I was shocked that I might once have thought this was OK.

All of these experiences generated a subterranean shift in my medical being. I started to see my doctor self much more clearly. I saw that I was doctoring from a position of professional expertosis, in a consulting room which was *my* room, with my things, photos of my children, snaps and souvenirs from my happy life. I came to see that the room itself demands the patient tell their story in a particular way.

I realised that a medical encounter is a ritualised performance in which I invite my patient to sit on a slightly inferior chair with a view of my framed qualifications. I have my props, medical instruments I use to examine and magnify and light up the patient's dis-ease. My shelves are stacked with the trappings of expertosis: texts dedicated to pattern recognition, pads of tick boxes, clinical guidelines, plastic-coated flow charts. The patient sees all these things, understands the unspoken rules of engagement.

I saw that medicine had trained me to hear the patient's story, then pass their words through an elaborate filtration system that analyses and discards, categorises and relabels, then finally produces a small specimen of manageable extract. The result is a sort of histological gaze at human suffering. I can attach labels to each sample of extract. The patient sees all of this happen.

Under my armour of expertosis, my humanity is barely visible. I became a doctor caricature. People who have been violated are very good at reading the room and know when someone feels safe. They can spot a doctor who is inauthentic, hiding behind professionalism. They ask themselves, 'Is my story safe with this person?' They give the story that the room asks for. And no more.

Nowadays, in my consulting room, I am trying new things. I have taken down my framed degrees. I have put novels on the shelves. I recently bought a beautiful velvet chair for the patients to sit in. It is in the most impoverished place I have ever worked, the carpet threadbare. The patients can't believe the red chair is for them. That chair does more good than any prescription I have to offer.

I have now put the best of medical history-taking, diagnosis and evidence-based treatment onto a small hard drive in a box under my desk. I tell my patients the box contains a medical model. It is a model with incredible effectiveness but also serious deficiencies. We can open it if it is useful for us. But let's begin with your story through your eyes. With my armoury of medicine removed, I find I can listen with my skin.

I now see my previous expertosis as a kind of grandiosity. What I have discovered is that when I am less grandiose and make me the doctor smaller, there is space for the other person to grow.

When I talk less, there is more room for their voice.

When I know less, they are able to know more.

When I act less, their capacity for action grows.

When I hesitate with my expert interpretations of their suffering, I leave a pause in which they can make their own meaning, let their cutting speak for itself.

In all of that, I learned how to be a doctor by *being*. In the end, it is through cultivating a quiet, curious, open *being-ness*, a kind of nothingness, that a something can emerge. I have gradually relaxed, noticed things I had been taught to ignore, and I have come to know myself as the other human character in the room.

Occasionally I might offer some wisdom, be the sage along the path, but I am only passing on what I have learned from meeting many people walking that path, offering them succour, asking what helps.

When we walk that path with our patients, they teach us, and we become humbled. We, as doctors, become a person who is prepared to see the suffering in others, and in doing so we meet our own monsters and mentors and challenges. Our own story.

Pākehā doctor, Māori patient

Throughout my career the colonisation story has sat in the consulting room like a taniwha. I have muddled through consultations with Māori, awkward and unsettled, unable to decode what that spirit in the room is trying to tell me.

The relationship between a Māori patient and Pākehā doctor is not neutral. We doctors cannot hide behind objectivity or professionalism, pretending *we* are not there. *We* live in, and accept our privilege in, a colonised Aotearoa. A Pākehā doctor has their own questions to face: Who am I in relation to colonisation? How can I build relationship, share power and fairly distribute resources?

I am barely deciphering what Pākehā is. I was brought up with a strong sense of my Irish Catholic ancestors, colonised by the British, leaving famine in their homeland and experiencing enormous opportunities in the New World.

My childhood was in the deep south of Aotearoa; I grew up with stories of rugged pioneers struggling up great braided rivers to break in the land. At school we loved poi and stick games. They were like folk dancing, quaint and fun, but divorced from context and culture.

I can remember Witi Ihimaera's book *Pounamu Pounamu* arriving in our living room, 'Poi E' strumming through the TV, and the footage of Whina Cooper leading the land march across the Auckland harbour bridge.

By the time I reached adulthood in the 1980s I knew Māori were angry, and rightly so; the big Treaty of Waitangi settlements were in the future. There was a sense we Pākehā needed to do something different, learn the rules of cultural competence, understand colonisation.

I hadn't really been near a Māori world until I worked in Whakatāne as a junior doctor. It was 1989, a few years before Te Whare Wānanga o Awanuiārangi was established on Domain Road. Te Kōhanga Reo was in its infancy, and I sensed a deep unspoken divide between Māori and Pākehā, two communities coexisting but walking past each other.

My first Māori patient was dead. She was a very old kuia with a moko kauae, lying in a hospital room too small for her whānau, who were spilling out into the corridor. It can feel like a pompous ritual, pronouncing that someone has died when everyone in the room already knows it to be true.

The whānau fell silent as my white coat entered. I could feel their eyes watching me. I tried to remember the cultural rules I had been taught about tapu and noa: 'Don't touch her head. Wash your hands. Don't get it wrong.' I left quickly, not wanting to make myself too important or get in the way of things I didn't understand.

The next week, out the hospital window, I saw a battered station wagon ready to collect a body from the morgue. A fight was brewing. In 1989 we still did a lot of post-mortems. It was Saturday so it wouldn't be completed until Monday, but they were not leaving without that body, their koro. A crowd gathered, the police arrived, and I felt a sickening discomfort.

Later, as a GP locum in the Far North, I remained unsure of my ground. In a clinic in a remote kāinga, a kaumātua was waiting quietly with his carved tokotoko. The nurse told me it was a year since his wife had died, the exact anniversary. I panicked. How could I talk to this man about his grief? His first language was not mine and his beliefs about the dead and the living were beyond my Pākehā grasp. I probably tried a clumsy 'Kia ora', and maybe I performed my own ritual by taking his blood pressure.

I remember that kaumātua as still and solid and kind, as though he was ministering to me, although of course I would never have told him I had lost someone too, a brother. But he had that way of *seeing* someone else, though barely looking. Doctors don't like being seen. They like to hide themselves.

These days I understand that the white coat and the chair I sit in are symbols of power and that building relationship from a place of power requires some dressing down and opening up of self.

Back then I thought that treating Māori like everyone else, with respect, curiosity, humility and honesty, was all I needed to do. But I know that is not enough, because frequently in consultations with Māori I get to the end and I do not have a clue what it was really about. I'm pretty good in my direct-questioning Pākehā way at getting to the crux of the matter. Pākehā patients tell me things because I know how to make it safe, make them trust me.

But often with Māori, my direct, upfront questioning seems to hit something solid and silent, and I know I have gone about it the wrong way, stumbling around seeking the cultural co-ordinates. Sometimes self-deprecating humour helps but mostly I have to start again, go back around to relationship, reposition myself, hold myself differently. I wonder now if this circuitous going back around is teaching me about a kōrero, a slower, softer way of revealing.

It is the whakamā patients I find the hardest. Their quiet, ashamed shyness discomforts me because whakamā feels like the embodiment of colonisation, and I want it to be not like that, but even that thought can make me bumble around being too loud and over-sized for the patient, whose personhood had been so diminished by the forces of history.

+

Later I worked in another rural clinic for a Māori health provider. One evening a very dignified wahine climbed into the rusted caravan that was my consulting room. She said she couldn't see very well. I was having trouble seeing myself because the caravan was very dimly lit. She wasn't forthcoming, and my questions seemed to bounce off her, back to me, without an answer.

How long? Blurry? Double vision? Wiggly lines? Pain? Medications? Other health problems? Red flags? The only flag was the colonising flag of Western medicine, which propelled me to take her story of *not seeing* and turn it into a medical story that made sense to me.

I had little to go on, so I took a blood sugar and shone a light in her eyes. I had no eye chart, and the caravan was too dim to see one anyway, so I suggested an optometrist. She looked past me, then to her feet. I pressed on, explaining what an optometrist was, assuming she didn't know, and at the same time aware I was assuming. Still nothing.

I was starting to feel silly. I didn't have a clue how to navigate this sea so I brought in the Māori support worker, who arranged to take her to the optometrist. The patient seemed grateful.

She never went. I don't know what she couldn't see. I suspect she didn't come about her eyes at all. But I do recall the gentle rock of that caravan as she stepped out of it into the night, as if the structure that held me was unsteady, with only a tentative footing on the whenua beneath.

+

Since then, I have learned about whakawhanaungatanga. Maybe in that caravan, I needed a very long word to reach across the divide between her brown eyes and my white optometrist. We are told whakawhanaungatanga means establishing connection. I've started asking where people are from, perhaps their iwi or home marae. Sometimes I know the area from a camping holiday or someone's farm, and sometimes that tenuous connection flicks a switch and there is a smile, and maybe the patient and I are now circling around each other in a way that seems to work, although I remain unsure exactly what made that happen.

More recently, on a normal day, in an iwi-run clinic, I greeted a new Māori patient, a bright-eyed woman, barefoot and toothless. All I said was 'Kia ora, Ripeka' and she bounced up, exclaiming, 'This is going to be a good consultation.'

I was dumbfounded. 'How do you know that?' I laughed, slightly nervous I might disappoint once I settled into my doctor's seat.

'I can just tell.'

Something had just happened. Maybe whakawhanaungatanga is simply a sensing or, as my friend Mere says, looking with your heart.

For a long time, my consultations were in the south of the country and most of the Māori I saw were far from their hapū. Their relationship with their whānau at home was not always straightforward. Sometimes they had left for a reason, for a life better than the idyllic one in my mind: of children growing up bilingual on a rural marae, gathering kaimoana. No, sometimes it was not like that.

I have also had many Māori patients who were adopted into Pākehā families. Often, they love those kind white parents, but sometimes it wasn't good. And some uneasy sensation passes through my trunk when I think of those adoptions; perhaps they were the 1960s version of the current Oranga Tamariki uplift of children, removing them from their families for their own good. What happened to those Māori mothers?

+

'Speak te reo, just do it,' says my Māori medical student. 'Stop being embarrassed or shy. It's an official language of Aotearoa.'

It's OK for him; he was brought up bilingual and he lives in a place where he hears the lilt and flow of the words every day.

If I start to feel self-conscious in a consultation, my te reo pronunciation is terrible. I have twice enrolled for a te reo course at Te Wānanga o Aotearoa and given up. In the middle-class south, the most te reo I heard was on National Radio. I'm making excuses. Maybe I'm a lazy Pākehā.

But now I have an app where I can hear the kupu spoken and I want to at least get pronunciation right, so I practise shaping those vowels with my ungainly Pākehā tongue. I have a lovely Māori patient who will sing a waiata with me at the end of our consultations. I'm not a singer, so between tunelessness and mispronunciation she has her work cut out.

She always explains the multi-layered meanings of the words; that the whenua is both the land we live on, the ground we plant in, and the placenta, and that an old woman can have a moko on her chin and the grandchildren around her bed are also her moko.

Over the years I have been taught the rules of cultural safety, but for me the rules needed stories and experiences to make sense. It's been the 'Aha' moments that have shifted the position of my feet on the landscape. Being Pākehā and middle-class, cross-cultural understanding was something I first learned about in university through an academic lens.

But it was powerful. In a single lecture in cultural anthropology, I learned that culture was much more than language, habits, ceremonies and stories. Culture was a cosmology, a question of where human life sits in the universe, in the great scheme of time and place.

I learned that place might not be just a point on a map, that time itself is a cultural construct and that place and time may be inseparable, bound by a sky father and an earth with personhood. And I came to know that our bodies may not be human machines as I had been taught in medical school but indivisible from whānau and tūpuna and wairua.

I recall that moment when I was pegging out my washing with my friend Tui, who was also my cleaner. It sounds problematic to admit the Pākehā doctor had a Māori cleaner, but Tui and I knew each other well from a women's theatre group. She was a superb cleaner. She told me over the clothesline that her mother and grandmother taught her to clean because it was important not to be seen as *dirty Māori*.

Tui's grandmother was so ashamed of being Māori that she told people she was Spanish: the shame of dirt, the shame of colour, the shame of speaking your own language. With a damp tea towel in my hand, I felt my own whakapapa of shame, back through generations of rugged pioneers right onto the deck of the *Endeavour*.

Maybe I didn't really get it in the way Tui did, but through all these experiences I was starting to get something.

+

In my final year of medical school, I worked in Sāmoa. My brother Sean's wife, Asimanogi, is Samoan, and I wanted to learn more about the culture: what I thought of as the language, habits, ceremonies and stories.

But what I experienced was my own culture. I came face to face with my expectations, my assumptions about how things should work and my ways of thinking about time and place and bodies. Until then, I had never realised I had a culture, because I had always lived in the world of the coloniser where everything works our way, seamlessly, for us.

Asi's uncle Leota welcomed me with lunch at Aggie Grey's Hotel, where he presented me with a copy of *Mau: Samoa's struggle for freedom*.[1] The book contained the horror of a Black Saturday I had never heard of, when New Zealand soldiers had opened fire on a crowd of unarmed Samoan protesters. I ate my soup with a silver spoon, at a colonial table, with a charismatic matai describing the scene where blood had spilt, just outside, in 1929.

I saw in Sāmoa that health is inextricably linked to world view and that medicine itself is a Western construct, with the power to colonise. I came to see that it might make more cosmological sense to suffer in the village under the care of a fofō or taulasea than to come to the hospital and die in the realm of the white man.

I had a strong sense of seeing in Sāmoa a culture only partially colonised. Cleaning obsession was not a thing. Land had not been 'sold' or stolen. We all believed, as we sang the words, 'We are Sāmoa, the greatest place of all.'

In Sāmoa I witnessed the power of indigenous self-determination, but it was many years before I heard about the concept of tino rangatiratanga or mana motuhake.

Before that I had to understand the Treaty of Waitangi in a new way. I remember the moment when someone showed me the list of Acts of Parliament that have been clear breaches of Te Tiriti. Not one or two such laws but pages and pages and pages of them.

An unclean story on a clean white page.

I am grateful for Te Tiriti o Waitangi. I feel lucky to live in a country where biculturalism is enshrined in the law, where there is a contract we have to honour, where every bit of health research or policy needs Māori input, where we can be held to account. Yet I know this is not enough.

+

Some time ago, I began working in a kaupapa Māori clinic run by a local iwi. We are trying to be whānau-centred, and my room has extra chairs, but they are often empty, as if the white coat medical model still has an invisible hold on the available mana in the room. It reminds me of the 'Aha' I had when I learned the concept of being mana-enhancing.[2] Sometimes when I don't have a clue, I ask myself, 'How can I build the mana of this person?'

But I still often get to the end of a consultation and don't have a clue. But I do understand that somewhere in the cosmology of being Māori the *I* is not as important as the *we*. So, when the *we* of the whānau has a problem, the *I* with severe diabetes simply stops their insulin to attend to the whānau.

I then see that my own idea of health starts with the *I*, with me: my health, my needs, my cholesterol, my important singular life. I bring my white middle-class sensibilities into the room, and I struggle to grasp why someone would just stop their insulin. My white coat wants to judge it.

In my head I hear those public health researchers at fever pitch about health equity. They tell me GPs are full of unconscious bias; we prescribe less allopurinol for Māori with gout than we do for Pākehā, and we are less likely to send Māori with chest pain to a cardiologist. I invite them into these consultations to help me, because it is really hard. I have no doubt I am full of biases and negative stereotyping but the kōrero is circling slowly and there is a taniwha in the room I am not quite seeing.

It was like that with another Māori woman whose blood pressure was 220 over 120, which is nearly a medical emergency, and I knew that no matter how much I injected my fears into her and urged her to take the pills, the prescription would not be filled. (Nor the other script to prevent her husband's gout.) I tried the motivational interviewing techniques I had been taught and she looked back at me, saying little. So I tried building relationship, presenting myself as someone she could trust.

I was still getting nowhere, so I resorted to humour, then negotiated one pill instead of four, then made sure she could get the script without a fee and offered the Māori nurse to follow up at home. I thought I had convinced her, but when she returned two months later, she had not taken any of my pills, nor had her husband. But they had been to the beach with their mokopuna to rest, and her blood pressure was now 170 over 90. It was still really high, but not life-threatening.

+

When I first read about Te Whare Tapa Whā,[3] Sir Mason Durie's model for Māori health, I did go 'Aha'. I took to the notion of health being bound up in the body and the mind, tinana and hinengaro, and I could see that bringing whānau into the room might help a patient accept my referral. But medicine does not have a language for the spirit, so I still get lost in something else beyond words: a feeling, a wairua that is wounded.

I tried with the beautiful Māori man who had been coming to see me every week. He had spent more of his life in prison than free, and had done terrible stuff to people, but he had also had atrocities enacted on him. He was semi-literate and in pain from long-ago injuries sustained while running from the cops. He lived in a decrepit boarding house and was lying low to keep out of trouble.

I had a very clumsy go at asking him about his spirituality and his pain. Weeks later to my amazement he said, 'Yeah, I think you are right about my pain. I've been talking to my mates in the boarding house about spiritual stuff.' He'd stopped his back pain medication and taken up gardening.

I think of him when I read about the Meihana model with its compelling image of the whānau and patient as the double hulls of a waka on a voyage to health and well-being.[4] It is a voyage in which the vessel needs all the components to be strong and seaworthy: the whānau and patient bound by the crossbeams of wairua, hinengaro, taiao, iwi katoa and tinana because as well as spiritual, mental, physical well-being is environmental and collective.

It is a journey that can be slowed by headwinds of colonisation, racism, marginalisation and migration. The journey can be energised by the ocean currents of tikanga, whānau and whenua, and by expert navigation skills, whakatere. The Meihana model gave me another 'Aha', helping me understand the multiple reasons why the waka may not reach its destination and giving me a sense of holistic indigenous ways of seeing.

I have had other 'Ahas'. When Tui and Wiki insisted our drama group had a kaupapa, a word I had never heard of, and that we practised manaakitanga with mihi, waiata and kai at our performances; when Mere took me to the pā where she lived as a child. With grace and humour she showed me her awa flowing under a road and her maunga covered in fancy houses because the surveyors drew the lines where they wanted. And she pointed out the hospital on the hill. Her people loaned the land to the Red Cross for emergency shelter during the war. It was never given back.

She laughs. 'It's funny. We told Prince Andrew about it, and he was going to talk to his mother. I don't know if he ever did.'

2.
System

System. The system is a colloquial and marginally disparaging term for the parts of the health service that involve rules, processes, funding policies, guidelines, quality measurements, institutional biases and collective paradigms with unspoken and unexamined assumptions. The practitioners often feel the system is out of touch with the realities of seeing patients and the system in itself can create farcical or even harmful outcomes.

A picnic in ED

I once broke my little toe. It was pointing sideways so I did a quick at-home realignment while my partner prepared a packed lunch, ready for an afternoon in the emergency department.

All the staff we met in ED were lovely. My toe was X-rayed and strapped, and I was put in a surgical shoe. The treatment was excellent.

But before all that, we had an interesting afternoon picnicking in the ED waiting room. I got to read all the signs. There were a lot of them: posters, notices, instructions, rules, values, warnings, bilingual spiritual directives, arrows pointing this way and that. It was a cacophony of words and symbols, but the biggest bold print said: *Our mission statement is caring for you.* (With *whakawhanaungatanga* and *manaakitanga* in small print underneath.)

I got the sense that the 25 square metres of blue lino designated for waiting was somehow dangerous. The staff never set foot on it. The receptionist and triage nurse were behind security screens. Orderlies managed to push wheelchairs back through to us without themselves touching the blue lino. Staff who opened locked doors to call the next patient in wore contamination gowns and didn't put a toe over the threshold. A very large poster read, *Your safety is our priority*, but I did wonder how safe I was in a zone clearly unsafe for staff.

We waiters improvised with our own support system. Mr

Bloody-Hand-In-Tea-Towel looked at my foot and smiled in solidarity. The son of Grandma-In-Dressing-Gown-With-Green-Handbag offered to get me a wheelchair. I had been standing on the red triage line for 15 minutes, toe throbbing, while the nurse took endless phone calls, each eliciting the same response: 'Yes, well, we are very busy', 'Yes, but we are very busy' and, 'Yes, 'cos we are very busy'.

While I waited, I checked if Weeping-Into-His-Fists-Bloke-In-Gumboots was OK. He gave me the thumbs up and went back to his weeping.

The All Blacks versus England test match had just come on a big silent screen, with teletext running along the bottom. Two of the players had names that sounded like 'daily' and 'care', which seemed serendipitous. I settled in, knowing that waiting in ED would be a game of at least 80 minutes. Plus ad breaks. Plus the expert analysis of the game.

Mr Dialysis arrived looking grey. We all knew he was coming because we had heard the triage nurse talking to the dialysis nurse on the phone. The poster over his head read, *Take the time to know your privacy principles.*

I was just reading the third principle when in came Miss Texas-With-A-Bunny-Ear-Hat, declaring loudly through the security screen hole that she had a pelvic issue. We heard her whole story while the teletext rugby commentary rolled along: *It's a recurring theme today* and *Care is going off.*

Several posters assured us that *We talk about domestic violence here.* I was nervous. Surely not through the hole in the security screen?

There was a children's play area with a locked gate. It was unclear whether the intention was to lock kids in or out. One wall was hand-painted with dreary fairies, there was a blackboard with no chalk and the TV screen said, *No input.* A sign over the emptiness said, *Please do not remove toys and beanbags from this area.* There were no toys or beanbags.

A notice informing us patients that *No photography or video recording is allowed* was quite near the sign that said, *Warning: This area is under video surveillance.* It's vaguely unnerving being under video surveillance. But the signs said so much about my rights and their care for me, I felt sure it was all in my best interests.

A noticeboard displayed the *Fast track daily performance table,* which recorded the number of attendees discharged within two hours. All the boxes were empty. It seemed I wasn't being fast-tracked because the rugby was into its seventieth minute and I was still waiting.

+

I'd finished my sandwiches and was feeling a little weary. The air was still and heavy. You could sense who had been waiting longest by their demeanour: recent arrival Mr Hedge-Trimmer was chipper and friendly, but Mr Hanky-Over-Eye, who had been there longer than me, got quieter and quieter and lower and lower in his plastic chair. I offered him half my banana. The hungry but unprepared resorted to nasty snacks from the vending machine.

Posters reminded us that if we had any questions we could call Healthline or 'Your GP' or even head over to the 'Urgent Doctor service' (if we had a spare $100). But the teletext assured us the All Blacks were holding on and I figured so should we.

A bad moment arose when Sick-Baby, Pink-Dressing-Gown and Limping-Man all arrived and were shuttled into the *actual* emergency department without waiting. WTF? But the referee's arm was aloft. The teletext muttered, *Tensions are rising.*

We all calmed down with the help of the little knitted teddy that stood on the reception desk, its smiling face pressed up against the inside of the security screen. I felt sure Teddy wanted to come out and play with us on the blue lino but *Infection control is our priority*, said the notice over the hand sanitiser.

The whistle had blown, English supporters had swung low coming to carry us home and we were back to reality TV. Mr Hedge-Trimmer was fast-tracked. I finished my crusts.

And in the corner a rather obscure little poster said, *Wouldn't you rather spend time with your whānau?*

Grandma goes to hospital

My mother was an early adopter of technology, so at 85 her cell phone is integral to her life. Thank goodness because she lives alone.

One night at 8 p.m. she calls. 'My nose is bleeding. It's all over the place, it's terrible.'

My mother doesn't say, 'It's terrible'.

She is at home, upstairs in her bedroom. I am at my home, 300 kilometres away.

She'd been in hospital the night before, also with a bleeding nose. She was given a very painful treatment and nose packing at 2 a.m., admitted by a house surgeon at 3.30 a.m., woken by the ward round at 8 a.m. and discharged home alone at 10 a.m. I think the hospital met their performance efficiency targets.

She is on dabigatran, a blood thinner.

'Mum,' I say, 'you need to set off your Independent at Home Emergency Alarm.' We had had it installed the week before.

'I have. I can't hear what they're saying. They're downstairs.'

'What do you mean, "They're downstairs"?'

'The box is downstairs in the cupboard.'

'What box?'

She's losing it.

I've never seen an actual Independent at Home Emergency

Alarm system, although I recommend them regularly. It is a little fraught getting the gist of how the alarm works because Mum is simultaneously holding her bleeding nose, speaking into her cell phone and answering my questions without her hearing aids. Apparently when she pushes the thing hanging around her neck it alerts the call centre, which talks to her through a speaker in a box, which has been placed inside a small cupboard by her front door. Her front door is along a hallway, down a flight of stairs and around the corner. She has a cell phone and a landline by her bed, but no one seems to ring those.

'It's OK, Mum. I'll just call the ambulance.'

'I don't want a paramedic.'

'Why not?'

'I had one last night. He was very capable, but he did an hour of protocols before even getting me in the ambulance. I just want to be taken to hospital. Can't I go in a taxi?'

'No.'

I ring her back. 'The ambulance is coming.'

'They'll take my pills off me in hospital. They don't give you anything until the house surgeon arrives.'

'Put a sleeping pill in your pocket and just take it when you get up to the ward.'

I can hear her giggle down the phone. I have unleashed her naughty schoolgirl.

+

Five hours later, at 1 a.m., she calls me from the ward.

'I'm all tucked up in bed and I've had my pill. The nurse says the house surgeon will be up to admit me in an hour or two. I'm just going to pretend I'm asleep.'

Good idea, I think.

At 10 a.m. she rings back.

'I had a good sleep. I ignored the house surgeon, and he went away again.'

At 11 a.m. she rings again.

'I'm stuck on the commode. I feel a bit dizzy, and I just can't get up.

'I've rung the bell.

'I've been here about half an hour.

'I can see them at the nurses' station.

'They can't hear me call out.

'I'm getting cold.

'I'm wondering if I should ring the hospital from my cell phone and ask to be put through to the ward?'

I ring the ward myself, gracious and polite. The nurses are over-stretched, I know that. The health service is over-stretched and seriously underfunded. I also know that if I want my mother looked after I need to charm them, engage them in relationship, thank them. Angry relatives don't engender kindness.

By 1 p.m. Mum is back home. Suzanne, her cleaner of 25 years, has picked her up and is making a cup of tea.

'Those alarm people keep speaking at me through that box. I have told them I haven't set off my alarm. I don't even want that alarm. I don't want them talking to me through a box. They have been ringing me and talking to me through that box for half an hour, telling me I am setting off the alarm. I'm not.'

I can hear the voice through the box down my phone.

'Just tell them you are OK and switch the box off at the wall,' I say. 'We can sort out the alarm later. Just settle in and have a cup of tea.'

Thank goodness for Suzanne, who discovers the alarm pendant is in Mum's slipper. The button was being pushed every time she stood up. But that's the end of the alarm. She's had enough. If she falls in the night, she will pull a blanket over herself and wait until morning.

A week later she falls in the night, slamming her ribs into the commode on the way down. Luckily by then my sister-in-law is there. Another ambulance, back to hospital.

My sister Shonagh calls in to the ward. Mum had an X-ray 72 hours ago but there is no result. For us the result is critical: if Mum has broken ribs, that means a whole lot more care is required for the next six weeks, and we will all need to rearrange our lives. If she is just a bit bruised, then we can get by for a week or so.

Shonagh, who is very warm and friendly, approaches a nurse. 'We were just wondering about her X-ray result?'

'She has broken ribs.'

'So, is that one rib or more than one?'

'I said ribzzzz.'

Our mission statement is caring for you, beams the sign on the wall.

(It turns out she didn't have broken ribs at all.)

Balint groups for patients

Decades ago, the British-Hungarian psychoanalyst Michael Balint started support groups for GPs where they could seek to understand challenging encounters with their patients. Once a month on a Friday morning I meet my lovely group of GPs and therapists, and we sit in a well-spaced circle and discuss tricky patients called *cases* in a Balint process that is both collegial and creative, and helps us process some of the more difficult patient interactions we have. My partner refers to my Balint group as my playgroup.

I have been thinking that patients often have distressing or perplexing interactions with doctors, so maybe patients could have Balint groups too. A patient might present a case like this.

'It was Friday afternoon, and I needed a script for my diabetic pill, Metformin. I was lucky to get an appointment at all, but when I heard the doctor's name my heart sank. To be honest, with all of life going on, you know, my recent separation and my mother's dementia, it was aggravating to have to go at all. So, to make my seventy-five dollars worthwhile, I made a wee list of other things to ask.

'I arrived early at 2.22 p.m. for my 2.30 p.m. appointment and was told by a snippety receptionist that I was seven minutes late for my 2.15 p.m. appointment. I knew I was right, but she insisted she was right. I felt somewhat like a naughty girl, but I knew I needed to be good if I wanted that prescription.

'She consulted the GP, who was walking out of the tearoom eating a cream bun. I could see them out the corner of my eye under the *Caring for You* practice logo.

'He agreed to see me for a quick visit, then proceeded to consult his computer. He suggested I could do with losing ten kilograms and I looked at him and thought, you could do with losing twenty, but I didn't say anything. I mentioned my list, but he said we had no time for a list due to my lateness. I would have to rebook.

'He then proceeded with his own list; took my blood pressure, which is always low, told me my blood results, which I had already seen, and said I needed a flu vaccine, which I had had at the pharmacy last week. I wasn't going to tell him that.

'Stupidly I volunteered that I had been a little stressed. I say stupidly because he seemed sort of encumbered and disconnected. The feeling in the room was a little unsafe. In any event he took no notice. After a lot of keyboard tapping he told the computer monitor he was increasing my dose of Metformin because my diabetic control wasn't good enough. I didn't tell him I already had diarrhoea from the amount I was on. Instead, I took the script for more with no intention of increasing it. It was as though he needed me to take it, to make him feel better.

'There was no way out except past the receptionist holding her EFTPOS machine. For some reason I found myself thanking her for fitting me in.'

+

The patient presenting their case now moves their chair back slightly and listens. The facilitators ensure the discussion is exploratory and creative; for example, 'What might be going on here, what might it be like to be this doctor or this patient?'

It is important the group does not offer advice or stray too far into their own stories of difficult consultations.

Her fellow patients might make these sorts of observations.

'Listening, I felt de-energised and hopeless.'

'My gut is churning. I think the feeling is rage.'

'I wanted to scream at the doctor, "Look at me, I'm here!".'

Or they might move into the psychoanalytic roots of Balint.

'Perhaps the doctor was weaned too early and is unable to form meaningful attachments?'

'Perhaps the doctor is re-enacting his position as an older sibling in a house run by an absent autocratic father?'

Someone might add that they loved the patient asserting their power by being non-compliant. Or how well the patient had done to keep safe in the face of the injustice about the appointment time and the shaming effect of the reference to her weight.

After 15 minutes or so, the case presenter moves back into the group and can speak or not.

They might say something like, 'That was really helpful. I'm feeling really cared for. And I get it. If my heart sinks, I need to listen to that feeling.'

The session might finish with a soothing cup of tea, a bliss ball, and a chat about real life.

Diabetes management: Evidence-based guidelines

Medicine these days is ruled by evidence-based guidelines in which very brainy epidemiologist types analyse and synthesise all the relevant medical research and tell us, the practitioners, the best treatments for each disease. Although it's not black and white. Not all research is good, some treatments have thin evidence, and the advice changes as new research comes to hand. And, well, drug companies may play a hand in it.

In New Zealand these guidelines are called HealthPathways and they are fantastic for things like pneumonia or heart attacks or sudden loss of vision. Your GP just clicks on HealthPathways and up pops the answer.

It also works for preventative health — although the evidence for preventative treatments is even trickier to prove — so as a GP I spend much of my day convincing well people, without symptoms, to take lots of medications to prevent ill health years down the track. That was always going to be a hard sell.

Let me explain. You come to me feeling perfectly healthy but I find your blood pressure is a little high and then I decide to do a check-up blood test that shows you have early diabetes and your cholesterol is a bit high. I then consult HealthPathways, which might recommend you take three or four pills every day for the rest of your life because the evidence supports these pills producing the best long-term outcome for your health — not to mention two or three major lifestyle interventions, all for your own good.

The medical world is pretty black and white. 'Good' patients gratefully follow their doctors down the chosen pathway and achieve all the required treatment goals. 'Bad' patients stand at the start of the pathway going, 'Yeah, nah', or take shortcuts or give up or just have other priorities in their lives or don't listen or lack grit and determination or are inexplicably non-compliant or just don't care about their health. Bad patients make the doctor's job difficult and reduce the poor doctor's score on the outcome performance standard called 'How well controlled are the diabetic patients in your practice?'

Doctors like good patients. But sadly, many patients are bad. HealthPathways meeting real life was always going to create some tricky conversations.

+

Take Gerry, for example. Three months ago, I diagnosed him with diabetes and sent him off with a diet and exercise programme and an evidence-based prescription. Together, we were going to bring those blood sugars down.

But three months down the track, things are not going well for Gerry. His blood sugars are worse, his weight has increased and, as he walks from the waiting room, he looks at the carpet, as if about to trip on some invisible hurdle.

I consult HealthPathways, which suggests motivational interviewing, so I ask how the diabetes is going.

He looks glum.

I move on to empathy to show I am on his side. I seek to find the barriers Gerry has to changing his behaviours so I can empower him to want to manage his diabetes and lifestyle more appropriately, with client-led achievable goals, through increasing health literacy and self-efficacy, and encouraging adherence to the achievable steps on the right path to good health.

He looks at his feet.

Out of the corner of my eye, I can see the 'smoking cessation' tick box on the computer screen. I want him to cheer up so I can get on with this and take his blood pressure and check his feet and get a urine sample. I have boxes to tick for all these things too.

I glance at the clock. Our 15 minutes are up.

I've known Gerry for about 10 years. He is a good man, in a vaguely unhappy marriage, doing his best, working like a dog to support his family.

I look at him.

'What happened?'

He stirs. He was too busy to exercise; his double shifts meant he could not plan his meals well.

'Sorry,' he mumbles.

The room goes quiet.

'Why do you need to work that hard?'

'Well . . .'

He looks at his hands.

'I suppose . . .

'My dad always told me I'd never amount to anything.'

I watch a big man cry.

There is no pathway for that.

+

As if the universe was trying to tell me something, the very next patient is Mrs Singh. A recent blood test shows she has diabetes and she is coming in for the results.

To be honest it's exciting for me to have patients with a real diagnosis as many of my patients have ill-defined complaints for which there is no medical explanation or health pathway. Today I feel like a real doctor.

I feel certain Mrs Singh will be a 'good' patient. I deliver my prepared speech for improving the health literacy of newly diagnosed diabetics. It's quite the soliloquy and it's going down well. Mrs Singh is nodding intently. I wind myself up. I have so much to say I can barely draw breath. I educate her, ply her with the pathophysiology, and reassure her that HealthPathways and I have the answers that will prevent the dire consequences of diabetes: multi-organ disease, blindness, leg amputations and early death. Patient information sheets and prescriptions spew from my printer. I am in my full power. It's intoxicating.

She listens politely. And when I finally pause, she says, 'Doctor Lucy, you see there is a small problem. For me it is not important how long I live, what is important is that I live my life as a good person.'

I put down my papers and smile. 'Sorry, Mrs Singh, we don't have a guideline for that.'

Smoking cessation performance standards

If I ask people whether or not they smoke and fill in that box on the computer, I get paid extra, and I get more if I offer smoking cessation advice.

It works like this. If I fill in these boxes for, say, 90 per cent of my patients then a magical algorithm tots them up and tells the authorities I am a good girl, and at the end of the year I get paid a bonus because I reached the smoking cessation performance standard, which is a good thing because we all know that smoking is a risk factor for terrible diseases and early death, and the more we ask smokers about it, the more likely they are to want to stop (smoking, that is).

Although because every health care worker in the land has a computer with smoking cessation tick boxes, every smoker is interrogated about it multiple times at every interaction with the health service, and I bet that's annoying and, frankly, having been a smoker myself at a young and impressionable age, which was a shameful thing but jolly fun, I think I would be tempted to just lie and say, 'Nah, not me, never smoked.' None of your business.

I'm also not sure anyone has researched the shame-inducing impact of these conversations. We have computer checklists to remind us to ask about things like weight and smoking and drinking, and if you are naughty these things are highlighted in red on your medical records. And if they show up red you will be asked about them multiple times, which can be so shaming you might decide not to go to the doctor at all.

So it's probably just as well we don't have a tick box for poverty or homelessness or the number of holes in your shoes, or whether you were beaten by your dad or raped by your neighbour. Anyway, we don't like to count things like that.

I'd like to get my end-of-year bonus, so I have been trying to get those 'smoking advice given' boxes filled in. It's not as easy as it sounds.

Take Eric. Eric is a grown man whose mother was murdered in front of him when he was 12. He wasn't doing so well when I saw him today. I asked him what helped. He said a good smoke. Motivational interviewing didn't seem quite right, so I asked him what else he needed. He said he was hungry, so I gave him my sandwich and took myself off to a café for lunch.

No bonus for that one.

Last week I visited lovely Sheena who used to be Steven. She is dying at home of lung cancer. I have offered her the best of things from my palliative care checklist: medications, commodes, night nurses, day nurses, meals on wheels, hospital beds, incontinence sheets, mouth cleaners and volunteer ladies. I have ticked the boxes on cultural and spiritual needs. I even came up with my own idea: a heater and a dehumidifier for her very damp bedroom. The nice ladies at the hospice shop were ready to help.

Sheena wanted none of it. But she had done her own client-initiated needs assessment, which resulted in me popping to the dairy to buy her a packet of cigarettes. My shout. And indeed, it was as if perpetual light shone upon her, early.

I was tempted to tick 'Smoking cessation discussed' but, really, she had end-stage lung cancer so does it matter?

No bonus.

Yesterday Tony came in with a chesty cough. He lives in a room with a single bed in an old boarding house. There had been a day when the city was blanketed in snow, so he had invited three homeless people to share his room, and he wondered if he had caught a bug off them. I asked about smoking. As if to reassure me, he explained they had all been on a butt hunt before the weather came in so they had enough butts to keep them going.

I told him how marvellous he was for bringing in homeless people out of the snow. I offered to give them all nicotine gum, because it might be cleaner than butts. He grinned as if I didn't know anything about anything, which is probably true, and said they didn't have enough teeth between them to chew one piece of my gum.

So I gave him a script for Fortisip, a nourishing drink to share with his guests. He looked so pleased that I thought he was about to jump out of the chair and hug me, and I confess that I was grateful he didn't because I had on a brand-new jacket, and he'd just apologised that he hadn't had a chance yet to go to the op shop for his fortnightly two-dollar bag of clean clothes. It's cheaper than the laundromat, he told me.

I felt as though Tony deserved the bonus for taking them all in.

Butt hunts are a thing. Spike told me last week his daily treat was picking up butts from the pavement and sitting in the gutter to smoke them, preferably after finding a good feed out of a rubbish bin. In case I ever needed to know, the butts outside the casino are always the longest. He was feeling a bit low so I decided not to go into smoking cessation.

Instead, I said, 'What else makes you feel good, Spike?'

He sat for a while. 'I like helping other people.'

But that's my job, I thought.

Performing an extraction using a Chawa Clip

I have been asked to do three Chawa Clips today. A Chawa is a Comprehensive Health and Well-Being Assessment, and Clip stands for a Client Led Individualised Plan. A Chawa Clip has exactly 212 questions detailing all aspects of the patient's health. It shouldn't be too hard because we have been given 30 minutes for each patient. That's one question every eight seconds.

We are told the Chawa Clip is a great chance to really engage with our chronically ill, high-needs patients so we can improve their health outcomes. Today I am visiting Daisy-Lee at home because she also needs a blood test, a flu injection and a mental health review. She has no car.

Daisy-Lee lives in a sleepout with a gap under the door and a two-bar heater. I am perched on the edge of an unsavoury chair. 'Do you eat 5+ veges a day?' begins the Chawa Clip. I'm editing already. Something tells me veges aren't a thing here, so I gaily ask if she's had breakfast.

'Yes,' but she's not inclined to tell me what she had. I move on.

'Do you smoke cigarettes?' She stares at the overflowing ashtray. I tick the box.

'Can you open your pill packs?'

'Yes,' she says. Yes, she always takes her pills, yes, she understands what they are for, yes, they are compatible with her health and cultural beliefs. Later, on my tick-box tour of her home, looking for hazards, I see them in the bin: unopened pill packs that had been carefully counted into little groups of days and times by a conscientious pharmacist.

'Do you drink alcohol?'

'No,' she says. But she is on thiamine, which is usually only given to alcoholics.

'Do you have any pain?' She hurts all over.

I press on hopefully. 'Do you exercise?' Daisy-Lee explains that she has both agoraphobia and claustrophobia, so it's best to just stay on her couch watching the telly. She hasn't been anywhere for years. I can't bear to ask her if she has been to a dentist recently, so I skip that box. I might have to make it up later, as the Chawa Clip has no space for unknowns.

She says she sleeps seven hours at night. She doesn't know if she snores because she has never slept with anyone, there is no one, they are all gone. There is no tick box for that.

'Are you stressed?' She stares at the muted TV.

My hand grips the clipboard holding the Chawa Clip.

I have been staring a bit too long at her overgrown toenails. I need to press on.

'Have you had any falls?' Just the one where she jumped off a building 10 years ago.

Noting the cue, I move to the suicide risk detection questionnaire, followed by the WENO depression score. It starts OK but I know Daisy-Lee is heading for a high score, which is bad. And I still have blood to take. Daisy-Lee is getting quieter, but I need to tick all the boxes to get the $100 funding, so I persevere with 'Have you been feeling bad about yourself, or that you are a failure, or have let yourself, or your family, down?'

Actually the truth is, I just couldn't ask her that. I just ticked

'Yes', which was possibly unethical but it wasn't the time to ask and the answer was going to be a long painful story, and I had 129 more questions to complete the Chawa Clip and make the claim. Which just goes to show the terrible dilemma of health care, where we are funded to do things that seem reasonable but in reality leave no room for what really matters if we really were client led.

+

I move on to something I hope might build relationship: a partners in health care score. Surely, we will be on the same page after this. I suggest she could read it and answer the questions herself. She says she can't read without her glasses and her glasses are lost.

It starts OK with 'Overall, what I know about my health condition is . . .' Not much, apparently.

I'm starting to feel like a prostitute paid to deliver services repugnant to me. I find myself apologising and I just can't ask question 152: 'Overall, I manage to live a healthy life (e.g. no smoking, moderate alcohol, healthy food, regular physical activity, manage stress)'. I mean, really, is this some sort of colonisation where the Chawa Clip now defines a good life?

'What gives you joy?' I ask. It isn't one of the questions.

'My cat,' she says.

'What's your favourite TV show?'

'*Survivor*.'

I ask her what would make her life easier. Also, not one of the 212 questions. She says new batteries for her TV remote.

I find myself offering to get her some on my way home. I know. No boundaries. But she is so happy when I drop them off.

Postscript: The Chawa Clip is my own invention but the process it represents is not.

Explaining the hazards of Cartesian dualism to the Minister of Health

Dear Minister of Health,

I think it's great that you are training so many mental health support workers. You have clearly seen the huge pools of despair in our country. We now have Health Improvement Practitioners (HIPs) and Wellness Advisors (WAs) and Health Coaches (HCs) and Primary Care Practice Assistants (PCPAs) ready to help.

However, GPs will continue working with mentally distressed people, as we have always done, and we are hoping you might fund us adequately for all these longer consultations.

Let me explain. HIPs and WAs and HCs and PCPAs are great — truly, I love the ones in our practice and so do the patients — but when patients bring their bodies to their GPs, they also bring their minds and lives and souls, and it is perilous to imagine a funder who whakapapas to Descartes splitting them at the door: body to GP, mind to mental health support and soul to chaplaincy service (but only on Tuesdays and Thursdays).

Let me explain by describing my day so you can see that any tidy reduction of persons into fundable pieces of mind, body and soul does not work, and that we GPs will be left doing what we have always done, moving freely between the physical and metaphysical, the spiritual and social body, and the pain and tremulousness of life, because we aspire (as your ministry apparently does) to holistic health models like Te Whare Tapa Whā.

We also know we cannot do the medicine well, or create your measurable and equitable health outcomes, without relationship. Relationship means building trust, and that happens when we respond to the patient's life, not just their body.

GPs are the only practitioners in the country expected to work with mental distress in 15 minutes. In reality we take the time the distressed person needs, run behind, then work unpaid in the evenings writing reports and ticking boxes to ensure we keep the funding we do have.

+

Today, a patient I have known for 20 years was discharged from mental health services because he is 'stable'. He didn't tell them he's telling his story to the Inquiry into Abuse in State Care. He is distraught, sobbing. He has chest pain and needs coronary angiography, but he is too anxious to get to his appointments. He doesn't trust state care. This is a 45-minute visit.

A young woman has cut herself. She comes for stitches. There is no eye contact, she doesn't want to talk about it. Suicide stats roll around in my head. While I close her wounds, I talk about cutting, why it helps, what it means. She declines referral to counselling but she does look at me. Her story will come out slowly over many tendings, to many wounds, over many months. Thirty minutes each visit.

A young man who is constantly suicidal is declined by mental health services, because he has 'emotional dysregulation', which apparently isn't a bad problem. I arrange his sickness benefit and disability allowance and medications and try referral to another service, which says the team will get back to me in their time, and by the time I have done all that for him he trusts me. And at the end of my day, he comes back with his two friends, and we spend an hour talking about peer support and I arrange a food parcel for them all. It is then he tells me he has such bad teeth he cannot chew, and could I check his ingrown toenail because he cannot walk. Total for the day: one and a half hours.

A woman is being bullied at work. She is sleep deprived from a waking baby and has a flare-up of her inflammatory bowel disease. She is hyperventilating. She is fighting previous alcohol abuse. Forty-five minutes.

A woman is living in her car, her ex-partner is a P addict, and her children have been taken into care. She is devastated. She desperately wants to change her life and get her kids back. I, too, am distressed; I have known her since she was 10. She is a good person. I give her a benefit form, some aroha and some hope. She has never had cervical screening and had rheumatic heart disease as a child but has been lost to follow-up. She says she will come back when she has money. Thirty-five minutes.

A young man who has been sexually abused comes for a sickness benefit. He is so anxious he can barely leave the house. He has stopped ACC counselling because it was too traumatic to relive his past. There is a 16-week wait for any other services. He is obsessively worried his anus is damaged and we are building towards the sexual health examination which will happen after about three more visits because his mind needs to be calm and his soul safe. He cannot pay for his appointment. Twenty-five minutes.

A young man has committed suicide. The GP who has known the family for many years visits the house for two hours. This is unpaid work.

A GP comes to me, burnt out. He says, 'I can't do this job anymore. I want to help people and I do, but there is no time, they cannot pay, there are long waits and I feel like I am holding them all.'

Warm regards, Minister. I hope there is a GP with time for you when you need it. And I hope they don't tell you that your tears are not their business; they just do body.

Are we uplifting mothers?

I looked again at the documentary showing social workers from Oranga Tamariki attempting to uplift a newborn baby from its mother. An uplift is a euphemism for forced removal of a baby because of concerns for its safety. In Aotearoa many of these babies are Māori.

The video is harrowing. I don't want it to be true. I like the story we all like, the one where our nation's social workers are doing beautifully funded mahi, supporting struggling mothers to care for their children and talking with whānau in a process overflowing with natural justice.

I think we have heard enough to know that story isn't true. But this is not just a problem of funding. It is a problem for all of us.

Since that video we have heard a lot from social workers, iwi, lawyers and politicians. We have heard from traumatised adults who were themselves uplifted as children. The people we have never heard from are the mothers. Like the young mother in the video, clinging to her new baby, they have been largely silent.

As a GP I have spoken to many women who have had their babies or children uplifted. These are grippingly distressing conversations. Without exception these women are extremely traumatised. Can you imagine the torment of having your baby taken, often without warning, against your will?

These mothers have been judged with vehemence on social media, have been declared guilty without trial. But the women

I have met are not monsters. They are our human kin, and they are hurting. They are women in circumstances that most of us could never imagine encountering. Some have been brought up in homes of poverty and violence. The uplift of their children can be a chilling re-enactment of violation and powerlessness. You can never unhear that scream of anguish filling a maternity ward; a mother with her baby taken.

What I hear from these mothers is an intense grief at the loss of their babies and a desire to do better. Sometimes the taking of children spurs them into action. They will do anything to get that baby back. Maybe they will leave the father and escape to the women's refuge, but they have no money, no home, no car; no resources to start building a life. They love that child, but they are on their own, stigmatised and untrusted.

The women I have met have very little legal literacy or any sense that they have rights. No one seems to be advocating for them. When I ask, 'What do you have to do to get your children back?' they look at me blankly.

I presume in my middle-class way that there is a process in which the reasons for removing children and the conditions for returning them are clearly written down. But no. Or if they are, the women seem to have no idea. Some tell me, 'I will never get them back.' Horrified, I think, how do you know that? How can that be true? Even if there was a risk to that baby in the first place, surely people can change, surely someone is helping you?

And when there are concerns about a baby, isn't that just the right moment in that mother's story to harness the best in her? Isn't that the moment to give her all the support she needs to parent, to get a warm home, and to believe in herself?

But no, it seems not. There is little funding for support. And yes, mostly that moment is lost, and the baby clothes stay folded, and the cot stays empty and the sight of them is so distressing to the family that maybe things don't go so well. And we might say this is evidence of their dysfunction in the first place. But I know if I had just given birth and my beautiful baby was taken away with no hope of return, well, I might go on a bender too.

There must be a better way. We do need to change our terrible record of child abuse. Children do need to be kept safe, but there seems to be no middle ground between leaving a child in marginal circumstances and irrevocably removing them.

The middle ground is where we invest in those mothers and harness that moment where they want to do their best. The middle ground is where we trust those in the whānau and hapū, seek out those who will do anything for the well-being of their moko.

This will not happen just by throwing an extra few million to Oranga Tamariki and hoping uplift statistics will go away. They won't improve until we all watch the video, see the horror and have compassion for those who have everything stacked against them, including the power of the state. I think we want to live in a country better than this.

The cost of cuts

A young woman is sitting in the velvet chair in my room, sobbing. 'I just want someone to help me. I keep asking for help and nothing happens. I need to know what is wrong in my head.'

Her referral to see a psychiatrist has been turned down because she is not 'bad enough'. She has overdosed twice this year and wants to hang herself. Emergency mental health services are swamped; they have sent her away three times without offering follow-up.

A Pasifika woman has had a continuous flooding period for six months. She doesn't meet the criteria for an ultrasound unless it is ordered by a gynaecologist, but she can't get in to see a gynaecologist because, despite severe anaemia, she isn't considered 'bad enough'. I have done all I can: medications, iron infusions, referrals. Intrauterine devices have fallen out. After months of bleeding and waiting, using all her sick leave, holiday pay and savings, she is finally getting a hysterectomy. The only way in was through the emergency department.

A man is coming to see me who has a rising PSA test for prostate cancer, but he cannot see a specialist because there is one urologist and no appointments, and months and months have gone by, and maybe it doesn't matter because he's not dying, yet. But I know if he was my dad, I'd pay for a private specialist because I can.

A woman has been waiting for an orthopaedic appointment for

six months. She has pain down her legs so severe she has to sit on the floor to vacuum. Now she has so much pressure on her spinal cord, she is losing control of her bowel. The only way to get service is through the emergency department, but it is too late: irreversible consequences have already happened.

I am remembering when my own mother had a catheter at the end of her life. I couldn't understand why her house smelled of stale urine. I washed the bags carefully every day. I asked the carer, who said it is normal for a catheter to smell. Then I asked the district nurse, who assured me there were no leaks. Then I rang the social services and was told they are only funded for one new bag every 10 days.

So I found a way to buy urine bags so they could be changed daily. The smell went. And I realised that houses stink of urine because people don't know how to demand something better, or perhaps they just accept their stinking lot in life and maybe their children need that four dollars a day to feed their own kids.

When I had young children, I decided not to get medical insurance for my family; I believed in the health service. When my son developed epilepsy I was grateful to the emergency department; grateful we got a CT scan on the same day he had two seizures. Although maybe that was because we were GPs, and the doctor's friend went to school with someone's sister. Other people wait months for their scans and maybe that's OK because they are not dying, just having fits. But I want you to know that waiting, even a day, to learn whether or not your child has a brain tumour is sheer terror.

I was grateful when we went home with the latest seizure medication and the promise of seeing a neurologist in one to two weeks. But the appointment didn't come for seven weeks, and he only got that one because I have a sense of entitlement, know how to ring an outpatient clinic, have money on my phone, have a phone, and I don't give up when I'm cut off.

Maybe a newly diagnosed epileptic is not a priority. He has only been given a life-changing diagnosis, where he can't drive or swim or work. He is only trying to reconfigure his life and identity, on a medication that is so sedating he can't think or study.

Maybe people like me should just pay more taxes, then move our families into the private health service. Because, honestly, I feel bad for taking up a space in that neurology waiting room, knowing that hundreds are queuing outside the door and down the street, backed up into the emergency department.

I used to work in a place full of people like me, people who could afford to pay or had insurance. Now I work with the hundreds of thousands in poverty. The need here is not twice as high as the need in Fendalton or Remuera or Wānaka; it is exponentially higher, not even on the same scale. We are swamped in need.

We are paid extra to meet performance targets for things like mammography and heart disease prevention, but these seem like middle-class concerns. We are worried about what our patients will eat tonight, how to get treatment for the crippling illnesses they already have, how to keep their chins up in the face of the most horrendous obstacles to a good life.

We care, but that is not enough.

Deliver us from the evil of inequity. Deliver something — we are desperate out here. We don't want anyone else to die waiting.

Equity and me

I keep thinking about that image depicting the difference between equality and equity. It is used extensively to explain why indigenous populations and people in poverty should get better-funded health services than those with less health need and greater personal resources.

There are three people standing behind a slightly decrepit fence trying to see a baseball game. The image labelled *Equality* shows the shortest person well below the top of the fence. *Equity* shows him standing on a couple of boxes, the proverbial hand up, so he can now see over the fence and enjoy the game.

It's a great image, and we get it — some people need more help because we don't start in the same place — but there are some disturbing elements. The three people are brown, and you get the sense that the white folks might already be inside the fence and not need a box at all. Indeed, on the other side of the baseball field we can see people sitting comfortably in a tiered stand with a clear view of the game. We can't see what colour these people are but I think we know.

Obviously, in an ideal, equitable world, we would invite the short one into the grandstand. At the very least, remove the fence, that great symbol of colonial division. But apparently, we are starting with offering a box. I'm wondering what needs to be in that box and who will provide it?

It is probably not for me to say what needs to be in the box —

it is for the small person to define what is needed. Perhaps my role is to say, 'I am in a position of power so I can help you get what you need.' Or maybe take out the middleman and just give the resources directly to the little guy. But that would require me and mine giving up our grandstand view and our control of resources.

Still, I can't help wondering what might be in that box. I'm prepared to be wrong, and I'm bound to be, as I have little idea what life is like behind that decrepit fence. The truth is I can't even see that fence from the grandstand because on my side it is hidden by corporate ads for new cars and luxury apartments and investment companies to protect my intergenerational wealth.

I do know that if someone tried to climb that fence and got over, the police would arrive and remove them. Looking over is one thing; climbing over is not OK.

My conundrum is that I have a seat in the grandstand outside of work, but in my work life I meet the boxless brown ones every day. We might even bond over sports results. So as a white doctor, what can I do in my consulting room to help fill the box that creates equity?

I suppose the first thing is not to see him as little. There is an inferiority and inadequacy in the word little. I might instead think of myself as oversized and him as just right.

I might imagine what it would be like to go behind the fence with him, sit down on the grass and have a chat.

I might even consider that he may not want to watch the game, that it isn't important for him. Perhaps someone else decided watching baseball games is a desirable, measurable outcome but in fact he has his own needs and longings.

But if he did want to watch the game, maybe he'd want to see it in his own way. He may not want to come into our grandstand at all —it might be more fun on the box. He and his people might want to build their own viewing platform and it might be very different to ours, better even. And maybe we could share some concrete and tools and knowledge of building and whatever else they need.

It is possible that he may not feel entitled to any of our boxes or indigenous-friendly grandstands. But if he walked away from our benevolence, we would be inclined to consider him ungrateful because we do not understand what it is like to be gifted a sense of being undeserving.

Which is why part of me wants to aim high, offer the grandstand with some manaaki. 'If you want to come into the grandstand I will accompany you. It is a foreign place full of rules and hazards and inexplicable ways of doing things, but we can navigate that together.'

But if we have to start small with the box, maybe we could fill it with mana, and maybe if I can stop being so self-important and oversized, I will enhance his mana.

Maybe I could help him load the box with his life experiences, his story and the stories of his people before him. Then he could stand on those things, feeling good and empowered, even if they weren't all happy stories in the grandstand way of seeing.

Maybe I need to fill the box with love and maybe my job is to find the love he has not experienced because he has been told so often that he is small and brown and inconsequential.

Maybe my job is to fill the box with respect because he has not experienced respect before from my grandstand people. And maybe that means I need to unpack my own judgements.

What I fear is that the box is simply aspirational. We hope it will appear, but we want someone else to make it happen: the funder, the health authorities, the social services.

Are we really prepared to make a difference? Will we ever share our tiered seats in the stand?

We can do better

It's a Friday morning and I'm driving down the coast to the Ngāti Toa all-of-staff conference at Te Rauparaha Arena. I am crying.

I'm listening to Emma Espiner's podcast *Getting Better: A year in the life of a Māori medical student.*[1] It is an exploration of Māori experiences in the health service, both as patients and professionals. But it is more than this; it is a vision for how health care can be better. How we can be better.

I am listening to a whānau from Porirua describing the lack of care they experienced when their father had a stroke. It makes my chest hurt. The realities of unconscious bias, whānau sleeping on the floor of the ICU corridor, the alien hostility of the health environment. It's making me weep, because I know we need to do better.

I am driving past the Ngāti Toa domain, where two Māori men were once hanged without trial. Past the mahinga kai of Pāuatahanui, murky with agricultural run-off. Over the harbour Takapūwāhia marae rests near the base of Rangituhi, renamed Colonial Knob by settlers who thought they had naming rights.

The arena is decorated for Matariki so the conference room is lit up with stars and lights, as if we are encased in a night sky waiting for dawn. I have never been to a health conference so inspirational. The energy is electric; ideas are flowing in a way that has been lost in the kōrero around health. The difference here is that this kaupapa is anchored in the people, improving prosperity and well-being, uplifting mana. These are the outcomes that matter. And the process matters; mana motuhake energises futures.

Helmut Modlik, the Ngāti Toa CEO, describes what holistic care really means. 'Any door people come through is the right door — you can't say "this problem is not my job".'

Earlier in Emma Espiner's podcast I had listened to Lynette Stewart, CEO of a kaupapa Māori health service. She is unequivocal: 'The first port of call is always whakawhanaungatanga and whānau.' Alongside her, clinical manager Sharon Russell calls on us to be our best selves because in health care for the dispossessed, we need to 'find the door and turn the light on'. I am inspired.

The next episode of the podcast features Professor Nadine Caron, the first indigenous Canadian surgeon. In her world view it is not possible to separate our professional and personal selves. I love this because I worked for 20 years in a small rural town where I was both doctor and me, part of the community. In many ways I think I did my best work when I was both doctor and known. Thank you, Nadine.

At the end of all that kōrero and an iwi conference under the stars, I feel hopeful that a new dawn is coming where something we have lost from medicine will be re-found.

That night, I drove a patient an hour back up the coast to her whānau. She had no car and I had just given her the sort of bad news that involves the sudden realisation of mortality, the telling of a story of a life through tears and tissues and laughter. And a smoke on the side of the road in the dark.

A few years back I probably wouldn't have put a patient in my car and driven up the coast past the historic sites on a Friday night, but I had Helmut, Nadine, Lynette and Sharon in my ear — 'Any door is the right door' — so I got in my car with the woman whose life I had just turned upside down, and we drove through the night, talking about our kids, towards her home.

A health care home

I keep seeing headlines about a new thing called the Health Care Home. Apparently it is a management strategy used to improve workflows in medical centres. But the name suggests something warmer and more welcoming to me.

I imagine a health care home with a riotous flower garden, the cuttings and bulbs donated by older ladies who know about such things. There would be a path to the front door, and to the side a yard with an outdoor table, a swing and a slide.

My imaginary health care home wouldn't have a waiting room, but there would be a large kitchen with a long table to sit around and a lounge nearby with a warm fire. Yes, people might wait, but this is a home so we also gather, share food, rest and do the stuff of life.

Maybe at the kitchen table you could buy fancy coffee but Pams instant would be free. Patients would be welcomed with hot soup in the winter made with unsold veges donated by supermarkets. And there'd be a plate on the table with a pile of little carrots cut into shapes for the kids.

Out the window of my health care home I can see people learning to plant a vege garden and digging a hāngī pit. And the kitchen would have a large fridge because for teenage boys, at least, the fridge is the central point of any home. It would be full of kai from the garden and people could take some away, just because, or perhaps in exchange for something they could offer.

The lounge could have guitars for anyone who wanted to strum or sing or join in. And there might be a sunroom where women could teach knitting or weaving with harakeke while kids colour in or have books read to them. And maybe there would be a room for prayer or meditation or any type of peace and quiet that's wanted.

In my health care home, the receptionist would not sit behind the desk; they would be on their feet, welcoming people. Well, if you insist, they could carry a tablet and update cell phone numbers and smoking status. The kaiāwhina in the kitchen would keep an eye out for people too.

The walls would be covered in colour and kids' pictures and photos of life. And maybe those living in their cars could have a shower or do a load of washing and hang it to dry on the rack above the fire.

I imagine you would see the doctor in a room with armchairs and we might start the consultation just by talking. And when the talking is done, we might stand side by side at the altar of the computer and do what is needed together. And there would be books and trinkets and a collection of tiny dinosaurs. And the examination bed would have a tartan cover and feather pillows, with floral lavalava and spotted curtains.

And there wouldn't be a staff room because a home contains a family. The staff might be more like your aunties.

There would still be an office, but the office could be like every office I have put in a home: on the south side and not a place you want to stay in too long because the kitchen table is nicer.

Of course, it's the twenty-first century so there would be free Wi-Fi and a recharging plug at every seat, and triage by artificial intelligence, and virtual consultations, and medical records secured by blockchain.

And there might be those wall stickers people have with

uplifting thoughts like 'Let's be kind' or perhaps a whakataukī: Me mahi tahi tātou mo te oranga o te iwi. We must work together for the well-being of all.

What else does a home have? Love? Yes, that's it. Unconditional love. For all.

3.
Doctor

Doctor. A doctor is a highly qualified authority trained in the diagnosis and treatment of disease within the scientific biomedical model. Doctors are well paid for their work and highly respected for their expertise. Doctors belong to a profession, meaning they must meet particular standards of behaviour and competence to achieve and maintain their membership of the group.

Narrating our selves

Doctors learn what a doctor is through stories. We learn how doctors ought to be, and ought not to be, through being in stories and being told stories. We intuit that some doctors' stories are silenced and others are honoured. The stories we are exposed to help us embody the character of 'doctor'. Over time we narrate ourselves into being by internalising stories that define our doctor self.

When we hear or take part in a story, we tend to locate it within wider narratives that help us create meaning. We might recognise medical narratives such as the Biomedical Brainbox, the Heroic Doctor and the Deeply Detached Doctor. These narratives are powerful in hospital medicine but can be problematic for GPs who need different narratives for how to be a doctor.

I love being a GP. I love the challenge of the uncertainty, the great mix of humanity, and the need to sit quietly with all sorts of problems of life. However, like most general practitioners, I suffer a bit from impostor syndrome, a vague sense that I am not a proper doctor. Perhaps it is the disconnect between the realities of my GP work and the archetypal doctor narratives I was taught in medical school. GPs don't often make clever diagnoses, sometimes patients have indecipherable problems for which I have no treatment, and I feel vaguely intimidated when I read hospital letters about things I have never heard of like 'CVKPD'. Even Google doesn't know what that is.

The closest I got to 'proper doctor' in my rural practice was during emergencies: rescuing an injured climber from a cliff top; alone after hours treating a woman with life-threatening asthma; a car accident at night in which a neighbour lies broken. These stories were part of the Heroic Doctor narrative, but mostly general practice isn't heroic.

+

On our journey to being doctor we started with stories from our culture, our families, our growing up, the Bible, the Qur'an, Grimms' fairy tales, stories handed down from our ancestors. These stories taught us how to be human, how to be good, what was important.

Before we got to medical school we had heard stories about doctors and about sickness. We had been patients. We knew about miraculous scientific cures, and we had probably absorbed the TV Doctor narrative. When I started medical school, doctors were like Dr Kildare: besuited white males who had good teeth and looked as if they were getting a lot of sex. Rugged diagnosticians with a kindly edge.

The problem for me was I didn't look like Dr Kildare at all. Picture this: 19 years old, 3 kilograms of wild hair, leather sandals and large bone earrings. I had been a teenager in the 'girls can do anything' era, and for the first time in its history my medical school class was more than half women.[1] But none of us looked like Dr Kildare and we never saw a woman doctor until our fourth year. She was a fantastic GP; pragmatic and kind, she wondered rather than knew. And she laughed. But stories about female doctors were rare.

The year I started medical school *More* magazine wrote a feature article about us, this curious phenomenon of the future, the female doctor. Alongside the article was a photograph of a young female model dressed in surgical scrubs with heavy make-up. The title of the article was 'Would you trust this woman with your life?'[2] Amazingly, in 1983, that seemed a reasonable question.

Even in 1995, when I joined another female doctor in a new rural practice, we were the first women doctors in the town. People rang and asked such things as 'Does your doctor write prescriptions?'

Luckily the feminists got it. Female doctors would understand hot flushes and period pains and provide hand mirrors for viewing one's cervix. The world would change. But back then the profession was in a gentlemanly panic.

'How can women be surgeons *and* have babies?'

'Doctors can't work part time and be any good.'

In medical school, the doctors were all men, so I struggled with what happened to *me* as I became a doctor. We also sensed an Invisible Doctor narrative in which our personhood was unseen under our white coats, so in some sense *me* disappeared anyway.

In a strange unconscious effort to make me visible, I took to wearing outrageous colourful outfits. But standing out was not enough. The consultants who taught us still couldn't remember our names or acknowledge us in hospital corridors. I can see now that the professor who could not see me was himself unseen. We were like two disembodied white coats walking past each other. There were only one or two teachers who were different — gracious gentlemen who quietly looked me in the eye, saw me and smiled.

Invisibility was evident in the feedback we received at the end of each ward attachment. On those single A5 sheets of paper, I was repeatedly told I was 'Satisfactory'. The options 'Very Good', 'Good' and 'Unsatisfactory' were always crossed out. That was it: one word. This reductionist, depersonalised correspondence was aptly called formative assessment.

+

The dominant and esteemed narrative of medical training was the Biomedical Brainbox.[3] We were immersed in stories of doctors who were very competitive, highly cognitive, expert diagnosticians, who knew what to do and got the dose right. We also learned that in the Invincible Doctor narrative, pushing on, working harder and longer without a chink of vulnerability was highly esteemed.

In medical school, the Biomedical Brainbox was drilled into us through a strange form of education called bedside teaching, in which a crowd of white coats gathered around the patient's hospital bed. The method was simple: publicly interrogate the medical student to the extent of their knowledge, then ask one more question just to humiliate them. We were learning from the unspoken curriculum: the shame of getting it wrong, of not knowing.

My medical professors still accompany me in my head. Occasionally they are useful, but more often they point out my deficiencies. 'Look at you now. Doctors don't swear in front of patients or crack jokes. You should know what the CVKPD is, Dr O'Hagan. You are winging it, aren't you?'

In medical school I understood that we needed to be something other than brainboxes, but I only learned the Reflective Compassionate Doctor narrative much later in general practice. In medical school we rarely saw kindness. Empathy was talked about, but we often took part in stories of appalling brutality.

The patient who was not in his bed for the ward round was decisively punished by a public examination in the hospital corridor; gown lifted up, testicles revealed and evaluated. The delirious old woman wailing, 'Help me doctor, help me doctor', as the ward round abandoned her, going off to do their important work. The man who boldly asked the professor, 'Excuse me, Doctor, I was just wondering what was wrong with me?' to have the white coat momentarily pause, switch back and bark, 'You've got cancer. Are you happy now?'

We were learning that the unspoken curriculum excused brutality so long as you met the Biomedical Brainbox gold standard, and that the Deeply Detached Doctor was the most effective doctor. These ward rounds taught us how to walk away from human suffering, to disappear from our own feelings, to detach from our intuitions and our bodies.

+

Fortunately, we medical students stuck together, supported each other, laughed, resisted. My friend Paddy and I spent a lot of the time crying in the toilets. We knew we could not cry anywhere else.

Recently, I met a patient who bore the most unbearable suffering I have seen in a long time: decades of physical and mental anguish. The patient was lamenting the loss of a previous GP, who had left the practice. I asked, 'What was it that he did that helped you?' After a long pause he said, 'When he did not know what to do, had nothing to offer me, I could see a tear in his eye.' I doubt he learned this in medical school; women cried, not doctors.

I had osmosed this idea of deep detachment by my third year, long before I saw a real live patient. Six weeks after my brother Sean drowned, I walked into my first ever post-mortem. In the lecture theatre stood a plinth on which lay a dead body, mottled and limp. The professor explained the young woman had drowned two days earlier.

I became motionless. I can still feel the violent roar as the circular saw cut through her breastbone, the blade slicing open her throat, and the pathologist excitedly showing us the critical evidence of drowning: that deadly mix of air and water, froth in the trachea. My mouth was parched. I was desperately trying not to go back to that river. And I knew instinctively that my story should stay invisible under my white coat.

A drowning

In the chill of dawn, we are alone on a riverbank. We have searched all night, stumbling, through wet black bush. Now, before us, is a vast brown flood field. In the mist, unconcerned trees and granite peaks just carry on with their eternal silent business. I know we will not find him. My brother is gone, pulled into that ugly brown underworld.

But still, his wife calls to him, 'Sean. Sean! Come home.'

I was not there when my brother went down. I did not feel the rock wobble under his foot, nor witness the moment his head disappeared. I did not see him briefly surface and gasp. I did not see, but I heard the story, and for many months I could not bear to make it end as it had: Sean struggling, the force of it, his backpack trapping him, breathing water, losing the light, desperate, and finally motionless.

In that pathology lecture I learned the unspoken curriculum: a doctor's experiences of life are not relevant to their work.

+

Later I was on a student placement on the psychiatric ward where my sister Mary had been a patient with recurring experiences of mania. I had been through those same locked doors as a visitor, but I told no one.

In the ward's formal assessment room with its huge pane of one-way glass, a psychiatrist would interview the new patients, who could not see the whole team gathered on the other side, observing them. Years later I recalled the sensation:

The Sunny Side

At 8.30 every morning, we gathered on the sunny side of
the one-way glass. We were us, *professional kin, dressed*
for dispassionate observation of them. *All untouchable.*

But I found I wanted to scream, to reach through
that impenetrable safety glass. For had not my own
dishevelled sister once sat in that observation box,
naked except for a green hospital gown gaping at
the back, revealing her soft, pale skin, exposed for
dissection, her unconsenting story to be surgically
excised, creating a wound they would kindly dress
twice daily, with Stelazine?

But I did not scream. I wept for my lost innocence,
and they saw my tears and they wanted to undress
them, kindly examine and excise them, categorise and
pathologise them. But I would not disrobe my story, I
did not trust their methods, for I knew how easy it was
to graduate on the wrong side of the one-way glass.

I was learning the Suited Professional narrative, one in which patients are *other*. Suited professionals don't have sisters in psychiatric wards.

In the Suited Professional narrative, doctors decide who is

sick and who is not, who is entitled and who is not, who has legitimacy and who does not. Professionals have privileges, a special relationship with society. We are trusted with public money.

To belong to the group, the Suited Professional Doctor must practise at an acceptable biomedical standard, observe professional boundaries and follow particular legal and ethical mores. We were taught the Suited Professional narrative in a series of cautionary tales about doctors outside the group: mentally unwell doctors, doctors who made mistakes, got it wrong, had addictions, burnout, who transgressed boundaries, fell from grace, became outsiders. This was the Shamed Doctor narrative.

+

Sometimes, even GPs need to be terribly clever Biomedical Brainboxes, but in general practice we can only make a biomedical diagnosis about 40 per cent of the time, most often of the common cold.[4] As GPs we find ourselves in very different stories from our hospital colleagues; stories without obvious answers, in which we need to take off our metaphorical white coats and just be.

GPs showed me the *being* of being a doctor. They were warm, enthusiastic teachers. Their way of doctoring was a revelation.

I read Ian McWhinney's *Textbook of Family Medicine* in one sitting.[5] At last someone was challenging the old narratives. Patient-centred medicine told us patients were more than body parts. Sickness was more than physical disease, the patients we cared for were fully human social and spiritual beings. Doctors themselves could be the medicine.

For doctors to be the medicine, they needed to ask themselves: What am I bringing? What is important here? Why are we doing this job? Later, when I studied medical philosophy and anthropology, we read the American oncologist Eric Cassell, who boldly asserted that 'the relief of suffering and the cure of disease must be seen as the twin obligations of the medical profession'.[6]

We have powerful biomedical tools that can, and do, relieve suffering: medications, surgery, chemotherapy, immunisations, intensive care units. However, we all know that sometimes the CVKPD doesn't work, or that the specialist was so rude to the patient that even though their affliction was cured, the experience itself created more suffering. Sometimes there is no CVKPD to offer and we are marooned and helpless, alone with a suffering patient. In these cases, we are left with, 'What is this person's suffering and how might it be relieved?'

I am reminded of a worried young GP who told me about a patient who failed to attend investigations for suspected bowel cancer. He described the patient as a lone ranger, a traumatised beneficiary, living in a boarding house, estranged from his family. Curious, he asked the patient, 'What is important to you in your life?' The man replied, 'I want to be able to give something to my kids that I never had. Perhaps some sport after school.' Our biomedical story is not the only story in people's lives and may not be the most important thing.

To respond to suffering we need our objective biomedical model, but we also need to be acutely self-aware, fully present, open. This type of doctoring is challenging because it means we do a complex crossover between extreme states of being: cognitive and intuitive, knowing and not knowing, or what British GP Iona Heath describes as 'oscillating vision', where we move rapidly and seamlessly between objective and subjective, science and story.[7]

+

General practice gave me a new narrative, the Reflective Compassionate Doctor. We were taught to 'reflect on and in our experiences'.[8] We learned by taking part in stories that took us to the edge of what we thought was possible for a doctor, trying things out, failing, then reflecting, trying new approaches.

When GPs relaxed and were themselves, it was powerful. But we were still uncomfortable with bringing *us* into the room, because the Suited Professional does not have a self. Patient-centred medicine implied doctors needed to be human but didn't tell us how to do this. According to GP academics Matthew Gothill and David Armstrong, it 'created a strange paradox . . . a person-centred doctor who was not yet themselves a person . . . a Dr No-body'.[9] We were still caricatures of Dr Kildare, just nicer.

The philosophy of general practice urges us to hear patients' stories differently, more fully, more compassionately, but still we hesitate to tell our own stories. We can tell our colleagues stories of failure, but only near misses in which nothing bad happened. We can tell each other about complaints, but only if the patient is obviously bonkers. We might mention a patient's suffering and our capable colleagues will point out the obvious things we have missed. For the things that really trouble us, the Reflective Compassionate Doctor is alone.

In recent years a new medical narrative has emerged: the Performance-measured Doctor. We are measured on our productivity and outcomes. Good doctors are very busy alone in their rooms, ticking a lot of boxes, collecting measurable data, the research evidence for CVKPD at their fingertips. In a grand collective delusion, we assume the things that are measurable are the most important.

There was a stage in my life when I visited my own GPs many times. I didn't have anything easily diagnosable, there was no pill to give me, no guideline. But those GPs were wonderful. They were kind, curious, imaginative and funny. We all knew how the doctor script rolled and could laugh at ourselves.

They accepted and held me in the mystery. What they did cannot be measured. They will not be rewarded for reaching a performance target or achieving required quality outcomes. Encounters like those are the essence of general practice, the work GPs do every day. Why do we not speak of it, value it? Why do we feel slightly ashamed that we are not proper doctors, measurable, detached, biomedical brainboxes?

Postscript: Sorry. I need to tell the doctors reading this that the CVKPD does not exist; it is a fiction. I didn't want to trick you but simply shed some light on our collective panic about not knowing.

Things real doctors do

I'd like to sound like a real doctor since I worked for 20 years in a far-away-from-hospitals mountain town and therefore I ought to have some heroic stories to tell. So perhaps I could tell you about the bus that slid off the ski field road, tumbling into the abyss, or the paraglider who dropped from the sky, or that small boy with a green cap who drowned under the bridge we pass over each day.

It being a small town, when an emergency call came we would always ask first, 'Who is it? Do we know them?', which I suppose is the wrong question for a doctor to ask down the emergency phone, but I had to know whether to steel myself before entering the scene because it might be my neighbour who fell, or my patient's husband hanging in the shed. And indeed once it was my own baby son who had gone blue after a coughing fit, and the babysitter had done mouth to mouth and then rung the clinic to tell us he was still alive but a bit limp, and as his father and I were the only doctors on duty, and the ambulance was parked just outside, and our home was 18 kilometres away, I knew the best thing to do was to grab that ambulance officer, who was also my practice nurse, and drive that oxygen supply to my baby.

I love ambulance officers with their crisp shirts and sturdy black boots and rank-bearing epaulettes. They were usually with us at rural emergencies, which is just as well because they know how all the blinking machines work. I mean every switch, every piece of tubing, every whatsit that links to another whatsit that makes a lifesaving gadget do its job.

Every two years we rural GPs had to do an emergency refresher course where we got to stick big sharp things into manikins, get rescued from squashed cars by the jaws of life and relearn the bits we had forgotten because in the last two years we had not actually seen someone with a gunshot or crashing heart failure or life threatening, chest-heaving asthma, but we knew that could happen any day, or more likely any night, when we were alone and far from help.

My life as a rural GP could be divided into the six months after an emergency refresher course when I felt invincible, ready for any sort of carnage, and the 18 months before the next course when I hoped I wouldn't be on call when the disaster happened.

To be honest I wasn't a very heroic rural GP, but I did get very good at staying calm and harnessing common sense in very high stress events that you might see only once in your career: a young skier becoming more and more unconscious after a head injury, a baby born at 24 weeks (thank goodness for rural midwives) or a young woman near death from internal bleeding (thank goodness for farmers in helicopters, who did a pretty good job before those big rescue choppers arrived).

+

We need refresher courses because emergency protocols change at a dizzying rate. For 20 years we have faithfully believed that 'thou shalt put a hard collar on anyone who has a sore neck and in whom the mechanism and velocity of injury could result in a fracture of the cervical spine.' This year a neck collar is an outdated blasphemy in the face of new scientific evidence. No neck collars are needed. 'Really?' Yes, really.

Emergency medicine is full of rules that later become blasphemies, like the golden hour, which I learned by rote and delivered with pomp and pretension as a young GP. 'If there is risk of shock from severe bleeding, thou shalt deliver large volumes of saline through two fourteen-bore intravenous cannulas in the first hour, to save the life.' Apparently nowadays this doesn't save a life at all but probably does the reverse.

Don't get me started on cardiopulmonary resuscitation (CPR). The ratio of chest compressions to mouth to mouth seems to have changed every year of my career, which leaves me in a continual panic: Is it 5:2? 10:1? 15:2? 30:2? Is it different for a kid? Is it different this year? Does it matter? Well, this year it doesn't, this year they tell us to ignore the airway and breathing in the first few minutes, forget the mouth and just get on with very emphatic chest compressions and defibrillation, and there is even a metronome on your emergency app that tells you how fast to compress the chest. Brilliant.

Emergencies in rural GP teams aren't like TV. There is no ER consultant standing at the end of the bed directing proceedings like a general. We stick to keeping it simple, no time for egos, everyone has something to contribute, and the person who comes into the room midway through the crisis will usually notice something the rest of us have overlooked. The best tool is the telephone, and talking to those wonderful ICU doctors who are so kind and say things like, 'You're doing well, have you taken the blood pressure?'

'Oh, yes, good idea!'

'And what is the patient's name?'

'Oh, no idea. Good question. We don't know them.'

On reflection I probably did save a couple of lives thanks to those ambulance officers, my nurses and farmers in gumboots flying helicopters, but some were not so lucky, and you never forget the sight of the freshly dead, the moment when the blinking machines get turned off, the life drains out and the family comes closer, like the father of the boy who had died despite our efforts, purple and blue with meningococcal sepsis.

That father. Years later he rang when I was on call because his wife had a pain in her chest and although he didn't say his name, I sensed it was him even before he said, 'I cannot see you. Is there another doctor?'

I did my best, steeled myself and found a colleague who, under the circumstances, was happy to get up in the night and help, and I thought I had held it together but as I put the phone down my body collapsed as if it didn't have the power to hold me up and I found myself face down on the floor, heaving my own snot and tears into a soggy patch on the carpet, remembering the sight of that dead child, the one we couldn't save, and thanking the good lord that my own baby son had been fine, just a little pale.

Rural practice

GP in small town

I have saved lives
but mostly I just watch lives
unfolding, as they do
I mainly give out tissues and condoms and tend the wounded
I am driven by curiosity
things are seldom what they seem
I have listened to the bodies of those who cannot speak
and heard the judgements of those who can
I thought I would change medicine
but it changed me
for better and for worse
I am the keeper of the town's secrets and the town's criers
and I put bandaids on

For two decades I lived in a rural town where I brought up my kids and worked as a GP. It was an incredible experience to live and work in the same place, and it was complex. As a doctor in a town of 6000 people, your patients also teach your kids, fix your car, do your accounts, live next door, play with your children and go to the same clubs, parties and community events. Patients even clean your house, renovate your bedroom and fix your blocked toilet.

In a small town this seems normal, but it's hard to explain that to colleagues from the city, who believe any self-disclosure is unprofessional, avoidable and extremely hazardous. It is definitely tricky territory, and it has to be thought through.

You cannot be 'unknown' as a GP in a rural town. It is very different to urban practice, where you most likely live and work in different suburbs. Patients have probably walked past my home and seen my underwear on my clothesline. My patients have seen my toddlers have tantrums; they have seen me dance in the pub; they have seen my teenager vomit at an after-party; they have seen me get changed at the pool; they have seen me fall over, get mad and cry. We are doctors, but in a small town we are connected into community, seen and known.

To avoid seeing patients outside of work, a rural GP could work an 80-hour week and hide at home the rest of the time, their partner doing all the out-in-the-community family stuff. But that was not appealing to me, and I didn't have a *wife*, so I needed to find a way to be both doctor and person in the same community. That meant understanding the nuances of boundaries and where the hazards were for me and the patient.

I did decline to put my home on a house-tour fundraiser for the toy library. The interior of my home needed to remain my personal, private space. Of course, patients who were friends, cleaners, builders and plumbers could come, but not random patients who just wanted a look under my bed.

Patients, especially in small towns, are alert to privacy breaches and from that assess the safety of their information. Early on, our practice decided privacy was paramount. In a small town it is hard to find a place where you can share your secrets safely, and for a medical centre to be that safe container all the staff had to adhere to very high levels of confidentiality. This boundary was critical.

We would not tell anyone we had seen so-and-so today if we had seen that person at work or even reveal that someone was a regular patient. We would not initiate a conversation outside of work with a patient about their health. Patients learned. If we didn't talk about medical things outside the medical centre, then they didn't.

It meant that the staff could have a life outside, relatively free of our medical role. It meant I could be out at a social event, standing with a small group, knowing the person next to me had an unwanted pregnancy or a newly diagnosed breast cancer or a suicidal son. We might exchange a look but not discuss it there. No one would even know they were my patient.

One of the problems with not talking to patients outside was when something significant had happened in their lives but you had not yet seen them as a patient. Maybe they had had a still birth in the city and you bumped into them at the petrol station or the supermarket. You desperately wanted to say something, but it wasn't appropriate to initiate that conversation in a public place. Best to smile, touch their arm, say, 'We've been thinking of you. I'll give you a call.' If they start to weep and ask to be comforted in front of the frozen peas, so be it.

+

This boundary also created some interesting outcomes. I ceased to gossip. I couldn't say anything about anyone, even if they weren't patients, because no one would know where I got the information. I did a lot of listening to other people's conversations, often about a person I knew from the clinic. I saw how quickly we judge without much information and without the curiosity to wonder what might lie beneath. Someone might call a patient a 'snobby bitch', but I knew she was overwhelmed with postnatal depression. Of course, I could say nothing.

In social conversations, I quietly listened and sometimes asked questions, gathering information about local people and families. I would sometimes hear things about a patient's life that the patient didn't even know: for example, their 12-year-old was having sex or their wife had just had an affair or their boss considered them to be a bad employee and wanted to get rid of them.

On the other hand, in the consulting room I learned from patients who was good to work for, which committees (and rural communities have a lot of them) were dysfunctional and which were great. I had a massive database of information that I couldn't share but that gave me a lot of context about the people I saw in consultations.

When you don't live and work in the same community, you can assume the 'patients you see' are the ones with the issues and the 'people you know' are normal people. I can assure you, they are one and the same. I was frequently aware of how the public self presented to the world outside was vastly different to the private self revealed in the consulting room.

I also learned about how stories change when they have been through multiple mouths. I could hear a story in the community about a situation I had been involved in as a doctor, an emergency, say, but the story I was told bore no relationship to the facts. I couldn't say anything. I got very good at nodding and wondering about the nature of truth. Sometimes I was told things in the community that made me wonder about the truth of the things I had been told by a patient. Truth is a fluid thing, and perhaps we are all putting out stories in a way that makes us look good.

Sometimes as the doctor you are the subject of negative talk because you did something that annoyed someone or got something wrong, and then altered versions of these events circulate back to you. Or someone might leave your practice without explanation, as they are entitled to, but then you run into them everywhere and you are back to smiling and nodding and holding yourself in some sense of integrity.

Another problem with living and working in the same place is that everyone looks familiar but you can't always recall where you met them. It was a nightmare being introduced to someone socially. I might be thinking, I know that face, have I recently looked at her vulva, or did I see her at school pickup? You can't say, 'Are you a patient?' Apart from anything else, it looks really bad if you have forgotten the consultation because they certainly remember it. I learned that the best thing is to smile, say hi, be very warm and wait for them to reveal where we had met.

+

I have been asked how I handled consulting with people I knew — my neighbour, my lawyer's receptionist, the school principal or someone I saw at a barbecue. The closer the acquaintance and the more complicated their issue, the trickier it gets, so it requires an alertness to my own process. I always got people to make an appointment, sit in the waiting room, pay and do the normal patient–doctor ritual.

The hazard is that you can overdo it or underdo it. Overdo means you get worried about getting something wrong and over-investigate or over-treat. Underdo means you bring some casualness into the room; you don't think it through and then you are at risk of missing something. You have to make yourself attend really carefully to your cognitive, diagnostic processes. Having said that, in many ways I think 'being known' made me a better doctor, less separate and distant.

Younger doctors starting out in rural practice have asked me,

'How do I make friends?' There is the potential for social isolation. It feels pretty safe to meet people in a group by joining a club or playing sport. People who belong to a church seem to have instant community. The people who are your patients in these places can be pretty relaxed about your presence, or they may ignore you and choose to step back.

To start with, workmates will invite you to social events where hopefully you will meet new people who aren't patients. Occasionally, a patient might ask you out for a coffee. As a general rule an invitation initiated in the consulting room feels all wrong, although I did once go to a garden club after being invited by an older female patient. I took a friend, and it was a semi-public space, so it felt OK.

But I wouldn't have gone to her house to see her garden because we had no connection other than the doctor–patient one. If she had been my neighbour and my patient, I might have agreed to looking around her vege patch. Likewise, my child being friends with a patient's child is a connection made outside the consultation room and so being in and out of each other's houses seems normal. But talking about medical problems is not.

It can be difficult for GPs in small towns to find really good friends. You can end up with a lot of close acquaintances. I only need one or two people I can share myself with. But I do need them. One challenge is that the people you might be good friends with tend to choose you as a GP. And fair enough, I like to choose a GP I have an affinity with.

If patients you know well socially only come once a year for something minor that is OK, but if you have supported them as their GP through huge life events or mental health issues, it doesn't feel OK to have them supporting you as their friend with your own vulnerabilities. Perhaps it is possible, but I have always felt that if I had been fully exposed then it was harder to hold the 'doctor' space for them.

Sometimes when people you have seen as patients start to become really good friends through connections outside, the best thing is to stop seeing them as a doctor at all. Although even that rule is problematic, because I have certainly been to after-hours emergencies where it was safer to treat a person close to me than to wait for another doctor to be found.

Perhaps an antidote to isolation is closer relationships with colleagues, keeping up contact with friends out of town and a good solid long-term relationship. Being single as a GP in a small town can be really hard. I also used professional supervision so I had some place to share myself. Having your own GP is great, but in rural areas your own GP will be your colleague and perhaps social acquaintance, even if you go to another town to see them.

Living and working in the same small community is a great learning about life. I think it made me a better person, less judgemental, more curious. I learned how to keep secrets. I learned that knowing another person is always provisional, that we can make up a story about someone else but should never assume it is true. It probably won't be.

The strange manual of appropriate professional behaviours for doctors

treating a patient's toenails with antifungals is appropriate
discussing one's own toenails is not

supplying tissues to a crying patient is appropriate
crying oneself is not

having clean teeth is appropriate
cleaning them in front of the patient is not

knowing what to do is appropriate
winging it is not

referring a patient with an obstructed bowel is appropriate
having a bowel oneself is not

following evidence-based guidelines is appropriate
listening to the feeling in the gut you don't have is not

telling a patient you like their shoes is appropriate
telling them you like their undies is not

pretending you know what you are doing is appropriate
admitting you are doing this is not

telling a colleague about a new herpes drug is appropriate
telling them they used the wrong treatment is not

responding rationally to a mistake is appropriate
telling your colleague you feel like a loser is not

implying to a patient that another doctor's treatment was not quite right is appropriate
admitting you did this is not

telling a patient to walk daily is appropriate
taking them for a walk is not

telling patients not to eat lollies is appropriate
offering them vegetables from your own garden is not

venting about difficult patients is appropriate
needing help to understand why they bother you is not

laughing about patients behind their backs is appropriate
laughing with patients is not

rolling your eyes when discussing a problem patient is appropriate
acknowledging the problem lies with you is not

putting a suicidal patient in a police car is appropriate
putting them in your own car is not

overlooking a patient's sexual abuse is appropriate
overlooking their high cholesterol is not

locking up an agitated person is appropriate
holding their hand is not

dancing at family weddings is appropriate
  dancing at the pub is not

saying oh dear is appropriate
  saying what the fuck is this all about is not

swearing is definitely not appropriate

Diary of an ill GP

I've been ill for a week. I know, doctors don't get sick. We certainly don't take time off work.

My partner says, 'You write off-work certificates all the time. You're always telling other people to rest when they are sick.'

Day one

I have earache. Real earache, like when you were a kid crying for mummy in the night. There is a cordless drill reaming out the side of my face but I still go to a Very Important Meeting with my Very Important Colleagues, then go home and sleep for five hours.

It hadn't occurred to me to take pain relief.

My partner, standing over me, says, 'Paracetamol and ibuprofen, you prescribe them all the time for earache. Take it.'

I wake with not a hint of ache. Shit, why am I pain free? Have I perforated my eardrum? Probably not — that only happens to patients. I get up feeling giddy and bump into the wall. I don't tell my partner because I have to give a Very Important Talk tomorrow and I don't want to cancel.

Bugger, the kids have used all the expired antibiotics in the house.

Day two

Now my other ear is sore. I give the talk, vertiginous and deaf.

I am worried I have a dead ear because I now have a whole new level of deafness, which, by the way, is vaguely peaceful. I already wear hearing aids because I've had cholesteatomas removed on both sides, so instead of real ears I have artificial ossicles and grafted eardrums.

My partner says, 'Aren't patients with reconstructed eardrums supposed to see a doctor if they have pain in their ears?'

At the after-hours clinic I pay $85 to see a medical student who is hyperventilating with anxiety because I am a doctor. I'm the patient but I find myself giving a teaching session on cholesteatoma.

I get Augmentin, which is pretty nauseating stuff, especially when you are already vertiginous. I nearly throw up.

Day three

I am too exhausted to see another GP for a different antibiotic. It's hell getting to a doctor when you are sick. But I find some unlabelled Maxolon under the seat of the car. One three times a day for nausea. I take two. Phew.

My partner says, 'You can't go to work this afternoon.'

Really? Yes, really. I catch myself thinking that even though I am too sick to go to a doctor, I'm not too sick to be one. It's so hard to text work and say you are not coming in.

What a hassle for the staff. What about the Very Important Patients with their Very Important Problems coming to see me, the Very Important Doctor? I send the text and sleep for four hours.

My partner yells, 'If a patient were as deaf as you, what would you recommend?'

Good point. I ring the rooms of my private ear surgeon, who is unfortunately holidaying in France. His colleague tells me to add in ciprofloxacin drops. He doesn't offer to write a prescription for it, so I have to text a colleague to write one as my own GP is on a climbing trip in Argentina and the practice won't give it to me without an appointment.

Day four

I sleep all morning. Maybe I'm just giving in to it. Wake up! You're a doctor.

My partner says, 'You're not going to work today either.'

Really? I send the text. I hear myself offering to come in for an hour, then retract it, and sleep for five hours.

Day five

I have muck coming out my ear. Perhaps my reconstructed ear is a mess with plastic ossicles floating around in the pus. I'm wondering about those windows I learned about in ear anatomy 30 years ago. Can they break? Maybe I should go back to the med student for another $85. Can't I just ring the ear specialist at the hospital? I'm a doctor, he will talk to me.

I try the private clinic. All I can say is thank the lord for lovely receptionists; they can make or break the illness experience. She fits me in tomorrow.

Day six

I am taming my bedhead in the shower so I look like a vaguely credible patient. I don't even have a bottle of pinot to give the surgeon and I don't have the energy to stop and get one.

But I do feel a bit better. Oh no, maybe I'll be wasting his time.

My partner says, 'That happens to us mere mortals too. We feel better by the time we get to the doctor.'

The Very Important Surgeon asks reassuring biomedical questions with a steely eye and conducts a lengthy ear toilette, which feels like a hot poker going through my brain.

But without a flicker of distaste (I hate to think what he sucked out of me), he reassured me he was glad I had come. Left eardrum perforated, right ear effusion.

Yay, it's a real diagnosis. I'm not malingering.

My partner says, 'You're happy you have a perforated eardrum that will hopefully heal? You *are* sick.'

Confession

forgive me father
for I have sinned
I took a cigarette at a party
and I inhaled
and it was good

forgive me colleagues
for I have sinned
it's hard to believe that in the 1980s
I shared an ashtray with a misspent youth
in the pinball corner of the med school caf

forgive me college
for I have relapsed
I took a cigarette at a party
and I inhaled
and it was good

how could it be
that a respectable
academic GP
with a wall of degrees
a fellow accredited to teach
could be sitting here wanting a cigarette
while writing an article for *GP Quarterly*?

a doctor obviously can't say yes
to the smoking question
cross to the other side
be one of those with a shameful health alert
which will trigger an invitation to confess their sins
and seek redemption
from a quick-quit practice nurse trained in
shameful confession, motivational penance
and conditional forgiveness

that is for patients

Today I want one of those old fella doctors

Some days I just want to see a young doctor. They are so uncomplicated. Their fingers are so quick on that keyboard that while I am still pondering what I might have forgotten to tell them they are writing me a prescription that has been passed quickly through the guideline and formulary filter with barely a pause for breath, and they have already texted me information for patients because they have been taught that even though I am a doctor I still need to be treated like a patient, and although I sense a little nervous energy because I'm one of those older doctors, they are so used to portraying 'professional', those young ones, that you wouldn't really know they were uncomfortable with me, just something about the relationship between the slope of the shoulder and the ears, or perhaps the quickness of their breath, gives them away.

Some days all I want is *my* GP, who laughs with me, who understands that I am a doctor like them, so I have already made myself a diagnosis and a comprehensive plan and we can have a wee giggle about the folly of that, and then my GP can look me in the eye and say, 'This is what I reckon', and I will trust them, because they are in their late forties, so they are still sharp but have been around long enough to back themselves and it will feel like such a relief to trust them that I will insist on paying for two appointments because that's how long it took.

Other days I want to go to one of those old fella doctors with leather shoes and a woollen jersey because they understand what it is like to live a life that started before there was colour TV or a worldwide web, but mostly I like those old fellas because I know they sing in the bath and because they have seen a lot of stuff, really, a lot of stuff, and when you've seen a lot of stuff you get an instinct for what matters, what just needs a gentle pat, what needs the tincture of time and what things are of the soul, and even though they may not use spiritual speak there is something in the way those leather shoes sit gently but firmly on the floor and the smooth rise and fall of that jersey that speaks to me, and I know something has been heard and things will get better, and I have it in me to work it out.

+

Today I don't want to see a random doctor I've never met at a place called 'Your Doctor Team Caring for You on Saturday Mornings' because I'm worried I might get one of those young men with a strut who have just given up their dream of being an orthopaedic surgeon because they want to do triathlons so urgent care works better for them, and I have a feeling they might not give me what I want, which is just a script for my cold sores, an antiviral tablet, preferably at the highest dose of 800 milligrams.

And I wonder whether other patients worry about waiting for two hours on a Saturday morning and paying a lot of money, fretting they will get a doctor who points out that cold sores are not a listed reason for taking antivirals and certainly not at 800 milligrams, and can't I see that the guidelines formulary filter is flashing, 'No, no, no', and isn't it his professional responsibility to follow the evidence and perhaps I could just go next door to the pharmacy and pay another $25 for an antiviral cream that I know doesn't work because I tried it in the 1980s, probably before he was born, and ended up with weeks of crusting, oozing, paining lips that made people want to social distance before we even knew what that was.

I am worried I will get this imaginary young doctor, and that when he has cornered himself with his 'computer says no' stance, I will have to either humour him or stroke his ego or give him a bit of older doctor to younger doctor banter to somehow turn the situation around to my advantage, so hopefully he feels vindicated in giving me just 400 milligrams that I will take two of anyway because I know if I get grumpy and say something like, 'Obviously you have never had cold sores', that will affront him and make him stand up, fingers far from the keyboard that could do that script, and to be honest it all feels rather fraught, especially as the reason I have cold sores is that I have had a huge week and I'm buggered, and really don't want to deal with the fact I forgot to get my script from my regular GP, who also gets cold sores and so, of course, takes 800 milligrams.

Today I just want an old fella doctor who will say, 'Sure, cold sores can be hell and you don't want to be going to a tangi covered in scabs, and how much do you usually take and, great to meet you, I liked the thing you wrote on bullying.'

Shameshameshame

We really are a strange bunch, doctors. The way we talk to each other. Or don't. We can seem a bit arrogant from the outside but really, we're just all mixed up.

For example, as part of our professional development we have to join a small group of doctors called a peer group where we share interesting cases and medical updates and general problems, in what is supposed to be a supportive collegial environment. But the conversation often rolls like this.

One doctor might tell the group about an interesting case of blahblahblah. Many of the doctors present have barely even heard of the disease blahblahblah because it is very rare so they feel a bit insecure and dumb but say nothing, while the real doctor informs them about the investigation and management of blahblahblah, implying they'd known that all along and hadn't just looked it up.

The next doctor might bring up how troubled they are by a patient's relentless pain and suffering, and another doctor will quickly chime in with the patently obvious answer. 'Oh, I would give this drug, it's new, with good evidence', end of conversation, and phew, the group avoided a discussion about feelings or anything uncomfortable, but in reality most of the group will go home and secretly look up the new drug because they don't know what it is but can't say they don't know what it is; and throughout this strange posturing all the doctors know, but don't say, that if a patient has such complex pain and suffering then the new drug probably won't help anyway.

By now half the group are feeling like impostors but one bravely asks their colleagues about a medical somethingsomething-something that doesn't feel clear-cut or easy to understand and one doctor will immediately know the answer and another two who know a bit about it will gaily join the 'know it all' group, leaving the impostors teetering.

One doctor might bring up a tricky somethingsomething-something and no one knows the answer. The room goes quiet. Someone coughs. A cheese and cracker gets picked up. Luckily by then the under-thirties have found the answer on their phones. Phew.

The good news is that the cell phone as the fount of all medical knowledge has somewhat democratised these sessions because the know-it-alls can be called to account by a quick look at the guidelines and the losers can quickly check they have it right before they dare to contribute.

+

It gets even more uncomfortable if one of our colleagues admits to being stressedstressedstressed. But the discomfort disperses quickly as the winners in the group give top tips on their superb work–life balance and clear professional boundaries.

And if you really are burnt out? Well, you probably wouldn't go to your doctors' peer group for support. You are more of a patient now. Not one of them. You could go but you might get comments like, 'You're not that bad are you, do you really need to stop work?' or 'I was burning out once, but I learned to say, "No"' or 'You'll be better after a holiday' or 'We all saw that coming'. (Which was very clever and astute of us, but we didn't know what to say or do, of course.)

Colleagues is a strange relationship. It has a sort of suit-and-tie formality, with no protocol or language for a situation where a colleague is struggling. I experienced this lack of protocol and language when I was the complaints officer in my practice. I had to respond to emails and letters from patients about things they were unhappy with. Talking to the patients about their concerns was easy, but at some point I had to tell the colleague involved there was a complaint about them, and that was hell. When is the right time to tell them? The beginning of the day when they will get upset? The end of the day when they will be exhausted and hungry? Delay and delay?

So imagine the excruciation of trying to relate to a colleague when something really very bad happens to them, like they get admitted to a psychiatric hospital or they make an error or the Medical Council investigates them or there is a death that might have been their fault. Generally we avoid that colleague and talk about them in hushed tones. We tell ourselves and each other that 'So-and-so is having some time off'. But mostly So-and-so just disappears for a while and is not spoken of again. Only it's a bit awkiesawkiesawkies when we meet So-and-so in the street.

I know some doctors are really nicenicenice and some of us are in peer support groups with doctors who are more like friends than colleagues, and some of us would send a card or a supportive text. But we all have these strange doctor-to-doctor behaviours in us, and when I catch myself doing these things, I feel a bit shocked.

+

What is all this weirdweirdweird behaviour about?

Here is my theory. It's all about avoiding shameshameshame. The argument runs like this. In medical school the archetypal teaching method was ferocious. We were humiliated for not knowing, for not coping, for laughing, for crying, for being tired, for just being human.

I suspect our early humiliation in medicine makes us shame avoidant so we have developed all these strange contortions and defences to protect ourselves from being shamed by looking like we know or looking like we're coping. This hiding of our reality (from ourselves and others) is sometimes useful because of course there is a time for appearing confident and sure and calm, but there is also a time for being honest. However, vulnerability is not part of the doctor persona.

I would argue that shame is just a form of social control and that the fear of being shamed makes us quite unconsciously conform to an external standard, the validity of which we haven't even examined. Is it really that bad to not know, to not cope, to make a mistake, to be vulnerable? Isn't that normal? Are these standards reasonable?

The problem for the struggling doctor is that they cannot be sure how safe they are sharing their struggles with their colleagues. We know we can be shamed by our colleagues. We have been.

We know our colleagues are sometimes not very self-aware, and we sense correctly that our distress might tap into their own bandaided vulnerabilities or their unconscious, well-protected childhood insecurities or their egotistical paternalism or their tendency to benevolent superiority, and we know that there is a risk their response might not feel that good. No wonder it is hard to ask a colleague for help.

It's a strange dance, though, between colleagues, because we don't really like to see another doctor shamed; it reminds us of our own vulnerability to shame. That's why it's so hard to tell another doctor there is a complaint about them and why we need to rescue our colleague with a simple answer. We see them getting close to a shaming event and we panic. 'Let me save my colleague from shame. I need to bring them back from the brink because I don't want to look into the abyss with them.' The abyss is terrifying. The edge is a no-go zone, even if most of us are on that edge.

If our struggling colleagues are beyond a simple rescue, we tend to get stuck, feel a bit awkward and step away from them. We might talk to each other about those colleagues, but we don't talk to them. We justify this by saying we have professional boundaries and cannot be our colleagues' doctors or counsellors or even friends. It's strange because we have all the skills to respond. We spend our days with distressed and struggling patients, but with colleagues we hesitate. Stepping towards our colleague is called peer support.

I've discovered a new doctor persona for myself as an unabashed over-discloser. I over-disclose about most things: the stuff I can't remember, my mistakes, my vulnerabilities and anxieties, the things that make me laugh and cry, my personal life. I'm sure my over-disclosures are deeply uncomfortable for some of my colleagues but there is also a sense of liberation.

And what I notice is that as soon as I disclose, others start to too. One honest testimony opens another, and soon we are all in a real conversation. That conversation starts with one doctor sharing one honest story about themselves. Without shame.

Burnout is always a long story

Looking back, I would say that I sort of unravelled. Over a few weeks, large chunks of my brain just fizzled out, the fuses blown. It was the weirdest feeling to be struggling to think. It was totally scary to realise I could not make my brain see another patient.

Like a good doctor, I pushed on, but it didn't work. It felt as if the main circuits of my mind had shut down and I was relying on seldom-used, weakly firing collaterals. I could switch on those collaterals and get through the day but they had no off switch, so by bedtime my mind was filled with an exhausted buzzing and I couldn't drift off to sleep.

It didn't feel like anxiety as there was no overthinking — my brain was beyond that. I felt physically drained, heavy in the body. I had always been a walker but now getting around the block was a huge effort. It didn't feel like chronic fatigue syndrome; I hadn't had a virus and moving my body didn't make things worse. It also didn't feel like depression, although the consequences were pretty upsetting.

I frantically read articles on doctor burnout, written by academics who didn't disclose whether they had ever had it. I was searching for a label for my experience, but no one described what was happening to me.

My GP listened with that intense curiosity GPs can have.

'You're right,' she said, her brow furrowed, 'there is no diagnostic category for this. It sounds to me a bit like a head injury.'

It did feel as if my head had been hit by some metaphorical blow and although the shutdown of my mind seemed to come on quickly, the forces that led to it had been there for many years. Burnout is always a long story. Being a doctor, I had an uncanny ability to push on through pressure, stress and distress, and keep going. It is both our strength and our weakness.

I am the kind of GP who gathers a lot of patients who are not straightforward. The biomedical model I have been taught does not explain what ails them. They have relentless pain, chronic fatigue, the effects of abuse, mysterious symptoms and complex mind–body overlaps.

I love this work. For me it is the most challenging and most satisfying. I like to be pushed to my own edge. Some would say that patients like that burn doctors out but I would say that these patients inspire me, teach me, enrich my life and make my work meaningful. Some patients take more energy, but the problem is not with the patient but with how we, as practitioners and health centres, respond to and accommodate their complexity.

General practice became harder in the 20 years that I was a rural doctor, and the complexity and demands continue to rise exponentially. The business of owning a practice is harder, with increasing amounts of measuring and reporting of outcomes. As hospitals become more stretched there is less access to specialist services. Some of the more straightforward work GPs used to do is now done by other health providers, so we are left with more complex and demanding problems.

The pressure can mount so slowly you barely notice it. At times I was probably teetering close to the edge of the abyss, as many

GPs are, but I felt confident I wouldn't go over. I was OK. Until life intervened.

+

General practice is a very hard job to do when your own life starts pressing down on you. The first thing that happened was the end of a 28-year relationship, the break-up of a family with two kids. It was a huge life event and the culmination of many years of exhausting relationship stress.

Something odd happens in a relationship that stops thriving. It's insidious, creeping up on you both over many years, permeating the fabric of your respect and care for each other. No one started it. No one knows when it began. It was as if we were a scratched record. We tried hard to change the track, turn the record over, quieten the volume. We didn't succeed. Increasingly we turned to other lives: my ex-partner to sport, and me to theatre and study. That worked for a while, but in the end a relationship is better if you share more than just your children.

I loved my family of four. I love the idea of family. I thought I could manage, but it became so tense that we were both being asphyxiated. We had years of trying to thrive in infertile, sometimes hostile, ground. It was exhausting. I approached 50 and looked ahead. 'Can I do another thirty years of this?' I asked myself. In the end I couldn't do it to him.

We were lucky because we were both ready to break up and we both wanted to recreate some sense of family beyond separation. My ex-partner is a very fair person so there was no meanness over money. We both had our own earning capacity and we had contributed pretty evenly to our assets. There was no one else involved. Even so, it was a monumental effort.

+

In a separation, you are untangling a very complex financial, legal and emotional knot, negotiating in the dynamic you are trying to get out of. It's easy to see how things can turn ugly and full of resentment, because sometimes you just want to scream back, dig your toes in, be righteous. I feel lucky this did not happen.

We separated everything: savings, mortgages, artworks, recipe books, kids' drawings, garden tools, bed linen, soft toys, empty jars. The bank manager was astonished when we came in together to sort out our bank accounts.

'Usually when there's a separation, one person comes in and the shared accounts are immediately frozen,' he said.

'Don't do that,' we replied. 'We've got bills to pay.'

At home we copied important documents and changed insurances, wills and family trusts. We carried on working together.

Then we had to tell our kids we were separating. It is the most unbearable thing a parent can do. We are hardwired to protect our children from harm, and yet this decision turns their worlds upside down. They don't want it to happen. We knew this was our moment to show our kids how to navigate the really difficult passages of life.

Our older child, a pragmatist at 12, said, 'Well, I guess it will be all right. It's a bit inconvenient.' Many years later he told me he had cried in his room. The younger one went silent, pale, as if his world had drained out of him. He couldn't speak for four hours, just needed either Mum or Dad to cuddle him. When he did speak, he couldn't understand it.

'You get on OK,' he said. 'It's just dumb. It's just stupid.'

Perhaps if children feel loved and cared for they don't notice the chronic discontent between their parents. Or maybe children normalise what they see in their family home until they grow up and experience something different. It wasn't all bad. We did great things as a family. We had a lot of fun. We shared a philosophy of life and parenting.

We had put all our energy into trying to stay together, so at the start of the separation, I was physically and emotionally spent. I should have taken three months off, but of course separation is a financial disaster so I thought I couldn't afford to. I didn't go to my GP — nothing in the culture of medicine told me that I needed to look after myself here.

We looked after everyone else: our kids, our parents, our extended family, friends and workmates. Everyone had a response, a grief of their own, an adjustment to make, a shift in the territories, an opinion. We did this together. We wanted to maintain the relationships we had; we didn't want people taking sides. It was really hard work.

Working with your ex-partner might sound stupid but, overall, it worked OK. In many ways there was less tension between us after we separated. Our workmates may recall it differently.

I did reduce my hours a little and I took less responsibility for practice management. I had a sense I couldn't deal with patients' big problems just then so I didn't pick up any clues about their distress. I was kind and polite and efficient but I didn't take the further steps I would have in the past — and I kept to time.

In the family home, I moved into the spare room. I had bought the house next door and spent two months renovating it while we adjusted to the new normal. The family home was on an acre and my new one was on four acres, so it wasn't too close. And just about then, something incredible happened. It was both awful, and beautiful.

+

I had a dream. The dream involved my best friend. But it was very short because I was desperately trying to wake myself up. 'That can't happen,' I screamed to myself, still asleep. And I woke up going, 'Oh, no.' And, 'Wow.'

Before the dream, I had no idea I had fallen in love with my best friend. I wasn't into women, and she still had a husband, and it was all too shocking, so I put the dream in a box under the bed and went about my life. But every few days I was tempted to open it and have a peek, and each time I was infused with the most beautiful and terrible reality.

Falling in love is beautiful — an almost psychotic state where anything is possible. I suddenly understood Valentine's Day and love hearts. Yes, psychotic. But it was also terrible. I had to tell her but I knew I risked losing her. So I went back to pretending it wasn't true. One day I was visiting her home and her lovely husband was making me cups of tea and offering to help fix things at my new house. It was unbearable.

'Lucy, get yourself together. You cannot be in this man's home when you are in love with his wife,' I told myself.

Lizzi and I had been friends for five years. We had done the most fantastic creative projects together, cutting-edge multimedia plays, homemade documentaries on challenging subjects, endless walks discussing the twists and turns of life. We saw each other most days. The thought of losing her was sheer anguish.

I'm pretty brave but I just couldn't make myself tell Lizzi I was in love with her. I had to tell myself, 'Well, if I lose my best friend, so be it. I've had an experience of being in love. It is a beautiful thing to have had even if it's not reciprocated.'

Finally, I packed a picnic and invited her for a walk in the hills. I could barely put one foot in front of the other. Still, I couldn't tell her. She told me later she feared something was up with me, that maybe I had a terrible diagnosis and was dying.

I went home and decided it could wait. She was about to go on an overseas trip with her husband and daughter. I had a house to move into. Another six weeks would be fine.

The next morning, I upended a full cup of coffee all over my desk. That finished me. We met at the lake, in my car.

'I have something to tell you.'

I couldn't do it. She was kind as always. I grabbed an old tea towel I kept in the glove box for cleaning up messes and I put it over my head. I had a whole speech ready, a declaration, an apology and a path for her to get away from me with dignity. I was so agitated, heaving back and forth, that my head kept hitting the steering wheel, setting off the horn.

'Just say it,' she said. 'It'll be OK.'

An hour passed and the car was getting hot.

'I think I've fallen in love with you,' I spluttered from under the tea towel. I was launching into my prepared speech when she said, 'Took you a while.'

Off came the tea towel. 'What did you say?'

Let me explain. I had fallen in love with a very gracious woman who didn't say things like 'Took you a while'. Later she said she had no idea why that came out of her mouth. It was as if all the tectonic plates of her life had just shifted into alignment. Clunk. She had no idea she was in love before that moment.

Yes, terribly romantic, but now we had a problem. She had a husband and daughter. I went home and read a short textbook on moral philosophy. I needed guidance. Was it OK to break up someone else's marriage in this way?

It was six months before it felt right to disclose our relationship.

The process was important to us. It needed to be revealed in the right way, at the right time, to the right people, in the right order. No one could find out accidentally. Some of them were not ready to hear such news. We had to wait.

Don't believe people who say having a secret relationship is exciting and fun. It's dismal. It's so dishonest and we both struggled with that. If it weren't for the psychosis of love, you just wouldn't do it. But the love hearts won in the end.

+

I'm glad this dream didn't happen before my separation; that would have set my moral compass spinning. However, part of me understands that we are on a continuum. If we are not nourished in the relationship we are in, then an unconscious part of us will look for love elsewhere.

The freedom of leaving a relationship and the delight of falling in love buoyed me for some time. But living with secrets is awful. I knew my good friends would know something was up, so I avoided them.

Through all this I continued working as a GP. I had been paralytic with fatigue before we made the decision to separate; now I could only do the patients and the inbox and go home. I kept the door of my room shut. I didn't want to chat or be asked questions. I lost touch with the practice. Maybe no one noticed. Maybe they did but weren't sure what to make of it or what to do.

My practice nurse and receptionist came in a few times to see if I was OK. I fobbed them off, told them I was fine, but I really appreciated their asking, and I felt cared for. Nurses and receptionists can be more likely to notice if a GP is not doing well. Colleagues can be too busy in their own rooms to see what is going on unless someone alerts them.

A few months after the separation and house-moving I got 'feedback' from my colleagues. I had been irritable with staff. I was a bit dumbfounded as I had little recollection of the incidents they described. It concerned me that I had come across as negative or disrespectful. I loved the people I worked with.

My only memory was how wretched I had felt internally as it was happening, how desperately I wanted someone to help me, not ask me to help them. In the end, I spoke to most of the staff about the feedback and they were kind and understanding.

I read this now and think, 'You needed help, a break. Being irritable was a sign.' But my ex-partner was doing OK, and he had just been through a separation too. I fronted up to my colleagues about my distress, but somehow there was no follow-up. I became increasingly isolated. I was probably hard to help, as doctors often are. Perhaps they talked to each other about me, but I was not aware of that.

Doctors are seldom good at supporting other doctors who are struggling, as if the struggle might be infectious. It's also hard for a doctor who feels like a loser to be helped by a colleague who seems to be a winner, but I do sense that if someone had opened my door and come in with a spirit of kindness, if they had not allowed themselves to be fobbed off, if they had gently pushed through my 'I'm OKs', I might have cracked. I didn't need 'feedback' so much as I needed kindness.

+

Soon after this, Lizzi and I revealed our relationship, first to her husband, then to my ex-partner, then to our kids. It had been an intense and demanding time; a separation, a new home, a new relationship. I was already running on empty, but I knew we had another set of huge life events before us and other people's responses to navigate. I had to keep going.

Lizzi's husband was understandably hurt but he is an honourable fellow. He was not surprised and painfully acknowledged that they, too, had grown apart. It was, of course, very hard on Lizzi's daughter. She needed time to adapt to the new normal, which was a catastrophic change, but she is a natural peacemaker.

My ex-partner, to his credit, was delighted. He has embraced Lizzi into our new version of our family and I am grateful we can stay in each other's houses, share meals and do life.

My pragmatic son said, 'Well, that's not really surprising.' Same-sex marriage had recently become legal and his younger brother was able to laugh when my ex-partner made jokes about who was going to give me away.

My mother, always a romantic, rang immediately. 'I couldn't imagine a lovelier woman for you to be with,' she said.

But it was another round of telling people, dealing with their responses and caring for those closest. Sadly, her separation was very difficult for Lizzi's family of origin and exposed some issues that were at that time unresolvable. She found me but felt as if she had lost her own kin. It was a terrible grief.

Now we had another roller coaster of separating bank accounts, mortgages, savings, cars, artworks, recipe books, kids' drawings, garden tools, bed linen, soft toys and empty jars.

It took 18 months of repeat visits to lawyers, accountants, banks and counsellors. And, simultaneously, we went through the elaborate process of joining our own lives: integrating kids, families and friends; sharing income, houses, bank accounts, insurance policies; creating new wills and relationship property agreements. Endless. But there was also a lot of love and nesting.

+

Many people ask whether, in a small town, a well-known GP getting together with another woman created a stir. To be honest, I don't know. Middle-class New Zealanders are a polite lot so they tend not to say things to your face. Apparently, we were the talk of the bridge club, but I only know that third hand.

I guess there will be homophobia in all communities, but the lesbian you know is always better than those other ones. We had both lived in town for 20 years and were well liked. A patient took my hand in front of the jam stall at the Presbyterian church fair, and said, 'I hear you have had some changes in your life. Good on you.'

Years later I met a young man from that same small town who told me that when he was an unhappy teenager, alone in his room, and heard his doctor had *come out*, well, that was the best thing ever.

At the time, we were most bothered by people placing us in the lesbian box as though we were now different to them, not part of their box. We didn't feel different. We had both just fallen in love with our best friend. The idea of being attracted to, or with, anyone else, male or female, was slightly abhorrent. We were in this one for life.

In retrospect I would say that it was strange being in a relationship with a woman in a very heterosexual community. We didn't realise this until several years later when we went to a lesbian doctors' conference and spent a whole two days free from the gaze of a heteronormative world. It was an incredible experience. We realised how much we alter our behaviour, instinctively knowing when it is not OK to hold hands in the street.

Separations and new relationships do create ripples. Falling in love changes us, frees us, and, with all our energy directed to each other, can alter dynamics with friends. They can feel left out. Perhaps some felt envious as they carried on in their own struggling relationships. But new friendships arose, and old ones were revived.

+

Two years after the dream, we had almost finished with the lawyers and accountants, and kids, friends and family were settling into a new normal. I felt as if I had been hanging on through two separations, and now life was about to get easier. In some ways it had been easy. We were in love, went on adventures, made gardens, read aloud to each other, giggled, danced and surprised each other.

After it was all done, we took a very long summer holiday. It was fantastic. Kids, beaches, books, long meandering walks. It felt like the beginning of the good bit.

I went back to work, rested and hopeful. But, about then, the unravelling started. Part of me watched my brain in slow meltdown, thinking, 'This can't be happening.' But I had seen it in others; coping through immense stress, then falling apart when the pressure came off. 'It's to be expected,' I had told such patients.

It reached the point where I would catch myself at 10 a.m. thinking, 'I just can't get my brain to see another patient.' Work felt like a monumental effort and in the end it felt unsafe to carry on in that state. I knew I needed to stop work for a significant length of time.

I decided the best thing to do was sell my practice. I had been thinking I might leave within a couple of years anyway, and I knew it would be really hard to rest when I still owned and shared responsibility for a business. It was possibly not the best idea to suddenly sell my practice right then. I didn't anticipate the grief that went along with it. Over 20 years, I had seen many people through difficulties and seen a lot of life. In some families, I had looked after four generations. I didn't realise how intimate these relationships were. I know intimate sounds the wrong word for a doctor to use. We like to think we are selflessly and professionally helping the patient, and we are, but we are also getting something back. That 'something' is profoundly intimate.

I didn't realise what those relationships with patients had given me until, overnight, I stopped work and never went back. I was immediately cut off from patients. I was not part of their stories anymore. I was still living in the small town where I had worked so I saw my patients everywhere. I wanted to hear what was happening in their lives but I couldn't really ask them in the supermarket. Patients would get cancer or die, or their children would suicide, and I wouldn't know.

I didn't have a chance to say goodbye, so I published a letter in the local paper:

> Dear Patients
>
> It is with great sadness that I am writing to let you know that I have sold my medical practice and have finished working as a GP in this area.
>
> I want to thank you for your support over the years. I also want to thank the team I have worked with. They are marvellous and I would trust them with my life!
>
> It has been a real privilege to be a GP in this community for 20 years. I have stitched many of you up, put plasters on others, helped you find a way through complex medical problems and stood

alongside you during births, deaths, marriages, break-ups, breakdowns and remarkable recoveries. I have seen a lot of life.

I have learned a lot from all of you: about being human, about how much more complex people's lives are than they appear on the surface, about bravery and resilience in the face of adversity. My own life is much richer for these experiences.

I know that sometimes I haven't been right, or got it right, for you, mostly through miscommunication or misunderstanding. For that I apologise.

(And sorry for always keeping you waiting!)

It is hard to go, but I know I leave you in good hands. My colleagues are all superb doctors with enthusiasm and energy. They are kind and compassionate human beings.

I will miss you all and wish you well as your lives continue to unfold.

Arohanui
Lucy O'Hagan

+

It can be fraught when doctors and other professionals leave partnerships. It's not something we practise for or do well. It was yet another separation, full of complexity and feelings. More lawyers, accountants and rows of figures that my frazzled brain could barely decipher.

After two years of being shut in my room, relationships had not been nurtured. And now I was leaving, there seemed no need to tend to a relationship with me because I was not part of the future. We did well to quickly negotiate and agree on the sale of my shares but things were said and done during my leaving that felt confusing and unpleasant. Perhaps others would say I had made life difficult for them.

To be fair, I was in no fit state to be going through another separation. I could barely think, and I had no internal protection against hurt. But hurt on top of burnout added significantly to my troubles and extended my recovery. It was a long time before I could go back.

I had lost my identity and I had a brain that wouldn't function. It would have been easier if I had planned to leave and was merrily going off to an interesting job elsewhere. Part of me knew I had the capacity to reinvent myself, eventually, but at that point, I was cast. I recall lying on my bed feeling that the superstructure of my self, what made me *me*, had collapsed; I had been stripped back to just flesh and bone. It was both terrifying and liberating. I was in some nothing space, a black void I didn't have the energy to fill.

I took to living slowly. Slow walking, slow cooking, slow housework. I couldn't take any stimulation. My beautiful friends Lynda and Jenny would ring me frequently, but sometimes I couldn't pick up the phone. Conversation was too tiring. I couldn't read or follow a complicated recipe or do difficult tasks. If I tried, my brain just shut down.

I developed a set of stretches I could do lying on my back with a wheat bag over my eyes. The darkness was soothing. I spent a lot of time on the bed, but from there I could walk out and sit on the veranda or meander slowly through our garden.

Our garden was a wild huddle behind a rose hedge. The veranda was still, warm and safe. Everything was close. I could sit near the family groups of parsley, spinach and dill nestled with self-seeded borage and unplanned sweet peas. Over the rose hedge, a grassy slope led into neighbouring backyards, the old church, the new school, the hall. Beyond that there was a long view across an agricultural moraine to the mountains.

I knew my burnt-out brain needed to huddle for a while, be near to life that demanded nothing. My burnt-out soul needed glimpses of that long view to know that something existed beyond.

My body needed to be slow, doing work but not with an ethic of work; acting not with a product in mind but with a stillness, just a tentative gesture towards something. That was enough for one day. It was an achievement to stand in gumboots, gather things for compost and scatter seeds.

+

I had planned to have a few months off, then start doing GP locums. But leaving the practice took four months, and by the end of it, I was in a worse state, so I had to take up my loss of income cover. I recall the first phone call to my insurance company. I wept. I felt like such a loser. The woman on the end of the phone was very kind and over the next 18 months we had monthly phone meetings. She played good cop, bad cop marvellously. She would be soft and gentle but then I would realise that she wasn't my mate, she represented an insurance company that wanted me back at work ASAP.

The insurer sent me to a psychiatrist. I knew he would be OK, as I had once heard him give a talk about his research into postnatal depression. The bit I remember is that his wife had suggested he was researching the wrong interventions. Her idea was a casserole study, asking, 'Do women with postnatal depression do better if someone brings them a casserole every week?' I got her point. I was rather in casserole deficit myself.

I knew I didn't have a psychiatric diagnosis and he agreed I wasn't depressed or anxious. In some great medical irony, burnout doesn't have a diagnostic category in that great manual of psychiatry, *DSM-5*. My cynical self thinks that is because burnout is the most common diagnosis in psychiatrists. After all, *DSM-5* has a diagnosis for everything: shyness, abnormal grief, sleep disorders. Thousands of doctors are burning out worldwide, but they don't suffer from anything 'real'. In the end, he said I had adjustment disorder, whatever that is.

The next week my medical registration came up for renewal.

+

I never answer calls from unknown numbers. I don't want surprising saboteurs in my day, not now. But I did pick it up. Remnant of good girl.

'Hello, Dr O'Hagan, it's Joy Burns from the Medical Council. We have received your online application for medical registration. But you have not filled in your workplace.'

'I don't have a workplace at the moment.'

'We can't process your application without the address of your workplace.'

'I'm not working.'

'Why do you need to be registered if you are not working?'

'I'd like to work soon.'

'Well, where will you be working then?'

'I don't know yet. I'm sick.'

'We still need the address of your workplace.'

'I ticked the box in section 9.'

'Section 9 goes straight to the health committee. I can't see that.'

I had ticked the box in section 9. I knew I would have to, but when I got to it, my finger froze over the 'Yes': 'In the last year have you had any illness or health problem that affected your capacity to work as a doctor?'

I ticked 'Yes' and wept. I knew what the consequences would be. I had seen it happen to other doctors.

Yes was like walking naked into a room full of suited colleagues for interrogation.

Yes meant I would be left in limbo, awaiting assessment. Some go from there to the slaughterhouse; some are allowed back in conditionally.

Yes was shame.

Yes, I do have a burnt-out brain. Yes, you might think it is a suspect diagnosis.

Yes, you might view me as some sort of flake who is probably just depressed or repressing her childhood.

But let me tell you how it is to have a brain that is pallid, without blood. Let me tell you how it is to lose your greatest asset, your mind, to not be able to think, follow a map, read or listen to National Radio. How dull it is to lie in a silent room.

Let me tell you how it feels to be humbled.

I did tick 'Yes'. I was well over the brink. Then up popped a PDF, all about what happens after you tick 'Yes'.

It was a dry, inhumane document, devoid of compassion, without a hint of care for the human being, the colleague who is ill. Not even 'Thank you for being honest' or 'It's really hard to tick that box but we are here to help you'.

No, it was an explanation of a formal legal process aimed at protecting patients from me.

Who was unsafe?

When I finally got to the Medical Council's health committee, they were very good to deal with. They decided that after five months 'off' I was now 'safe' for a gradual return to work. Ironically, I was probably a much safer doctor now than I had been in the two years before I unravelled. I'm lucky I didn't make a mistake in that time.

I had a restraint of trade so my gradual return to work involved travelling for an hour each way on top of half a day of GP work. I was very grateful to the colleagues in nearby towns who supported my tentative return to work.

I was so lucky to have Lizzi. She was so kind. She was optimistic about my future and my capacities. She was realistic about what I could do each day.

I was not realistic. I was frustrated. I didn't want to be sick. I wanted to get on with life and I fought it and denied it until I found myself back on my bed, exhausted. It was only Lizzi's acceptance of what is that allowed me to let myself be ill. She has a soft, quiet way about her. She never got upset or frustrated with me. For several months, she drove me to work, an hour each way.

In the year that followed, I gave myself a treat: part-time online study with what was the Center for Narrative Practice in Boston. It was fantastic. Full of ideas and interesting people. And in some strange way, because no one knew me, I could start creating a new character for myself, in a different story.

+

At the same time, I needed to make sense of the story I had been in, so I spoke to one of my former partners and one night Lizzi drove me into town to visit my old GP practice. We went late to be sure we would be alone. I surprised myself by weeping all 18 kilometres, remembering the many times I had driven that road at night as the on-call doctor.

It was a year since I had been back into the building. I went into what had been my consulting room and lay on the floor in the dark. It hadn't ended well. I wanted to see it from a different angle and sitting in the chairs was too literal. I needed to feel the cool concrete slab under my back, to let something mysterious and sore drain out through the beige carpet tiles, through the firmness, into the earth.

The wall the patients saw from their chair was painted a warm autumn tone called Karma. On the golden green I had hung coloured paintings, drawings of fearful passages and photographs of angels. My seat faced the other way, towards the sterile basin, hand sanitiser and eye chart. I had put a tiny image of an unhygienic Grecian urn above the paper-towel dispenser.

I remembered the procession of souls who had come in and out, in and out of that room carrying their bundles of troubles.

I felt soothed by them; their courage infused me.

They made me smile.

I had returned because I needed this room to talk to me.

I had crept back in the dark to feel the angels, hear the souls whisper to me and let all the rest seep out of me.

It was not the heat of their troubles that burnt me, it was the heat of my own.

Sleeping with the ancestors

We are on a coast road with million-dollar views, million-dollar houses, tidy curbs and gutters and clipped hedges. Around a headland the road becomes gravel, bush pours down the hill, the homes are simple and, by the beach, there is a wharenui.

I have flown north to a noho marae for a group of young GPs. I am supposed to be one of the teachers but after the humbling scarification of burnout, I don't feel so steady in my convictions.

I am sharing a ride from the airport with our kaumātua, who is in his eighties. He tells me with a giggle that retirement is a Pākehā construction. He will deconstruct many of my ways of seeing in the next 24 hours. I will learn that an older man has a place at a wānanga about culture and health; even if he shuffles a little on his feet and falls asleep in the middle of the kōrero, it matters not, because when he wakes at dawn, opens the doors of the wharenui and chants to the rising sun, I experience something not found in a textbook.

Before we went to the marae, we had visited the National Library's Te Ahumairangi, home of the original Te Tiriti document. There we met a famous Treaty of Waitangi historian: she is Pākehā, diminutive and gracious, the daughter of honourable civil servants. Smiling, in that way polite Pākehā do, she suggests we could just ignore the English version of Te Tiriti. 'It was signed in Māori, so we should read it in Māori.' *Of course*, we all think simultaneously.

She describes the Waitangi Tribunal as a revolution. 'May the revolution continue,' she smiles, leading us into the waka huia containing the original treaty document.

There is something profound about being inside a waka huia with a taonga, inside a carved wooden vessel with our founding document. A physical experience you can't get from a photograph.

Later, at the marae, GP trainees and teachers gather with our kaumātua at the waharoa, the gateway. A karanga sounds from the wharenui, and a wahine from our group responds, her voice channelling some other physical and spiritual dimension. I am transfixed. I meet her later, a young Māori GP, graciously challenging us to be pro-equity practitioners.

In the afternoon one of the aunties comes to speak. She's also an academic and knows about colonisation. She starts with the pre-European world of her ancestor, born before Cook's landing. She describes every generation that follows, colonisation picking away at a people, the loss of land and language, the ravage of disease, the cost of urbanisation. But ultimately, she tells a story of mana and resilience.

At the pōwhiri we have been welcomed by the whānau and told the story of this wharenui. The young people had had a thirst for a carved meeting house but to build it they had to learn the arts of carving and weaving and to do that they had to immerse themselves deeply in te ao Māori, in the tikanga and the language of their tūpuna.

We sit under those ancestors, carved into the backbone of the building. The kōwhaiwhai ribs, arching over us, describe our relationship with an earth mother, our interconnectedness to all living things and each other, past and present. Tukutuku panels tell us in symbols about the stars, the oceans, our food sources, the strength of a warrior, the love of a parent, the sacred and the ordinary in human relationships.

A Māori fourth-year medical student is among us. In this place she stands taller. Here she can speak. A GP registrar who whakapapas Māori with some hesitancy is embraced and something stirs in her. An Asian registrar laments how much he misses consulting in his own culture. Our kaumātua blesses the two doctors who are hapū and says karakia over a pounamu he presents to a Pākehā teacher. Incredibly, there are two Pākehā doctors who are fluent te reo speakers. Yes, there has been a revolution.

In this whare we can talk about the ancient art of medicine. We can say love and medicine in the same sentence. A GP poet weaves us with words until we know we too can be the medicine.

+

By evening there is a sense of exhaustion and excitement and sadness. As we lie down in the semi-darkness to sleep, I feel as though the carved building above and around me has seen my cracks but is holding me close. It makes me think that a consultation is like a whare, a space for hurt and anger and love, where the patient might come with their shell cracked and know that they will be contained, safely.

In the morning we practise cross-cultural consultations with Māori actors and it isn't so easy. These things are never as simple as the guidelines make them sound.

One of the actors challenges us: 'I know those Māori academics tell you to ask me where I am from. When a Māori asks me that, we are connecting with each other. But the only Pākehā who asks me that question is a policeman.'

I see now that GPs, like the police, are part of the power structure of colonisation. We belong to institutions that have harmed people. We need to do something different, to be trusted.

Our kaumātua brings us back, reminds us to look at the sea, honour the wai, marvel at the flight of the manu, listen for the tūpuna. He was brought up by a grandmother who spoke to and named the fruit trees. When she died, the trees died. It was both a mystery and not a mystery. He offers to show us Matariki at 3 a.m. He is always awake then, ready for the ebb and flow of night and day.

'Every morning I wake up and tell myself that this is going to be the best day of my life,' he tells us. He is a man of positivity.

And let me not forget in the grandness of our kōrero that we were fed. Women in the wharekai doing what wāhine in all cultures do: preparing kai with aroha. I am struck by the incredible generosity of the colonised towards the coloniser. Their manaakitanga is not a lonely word under a health care logo; it is showing us a path forward, an experience of relationship.

I am reminded of Moana Jackson, who reframed decolonisation as an ethic of restoration that is concerned with the balance of relationships. He writes: 'Stories for and about transformation rely on honesty about the misremembered stories and the foresight to see where different stories might lead.'[1] I sensed, in this whare, both disturbance and pain, exhilaration and possibilities.

It was unsettling but something had sunk into me. As I flew home to the deep south, following the mountainous spine of Te Waipounamu, the farewell karakia of the kaumātua soothed me: Kia hora te marino, kia whakapapa pounamu te moana, kia tere te kārohirohi i mua i tōu huarahi.

May calm be spread around you, may the sea glisten like greenstone and the shimmer of summer dance across your path.

The Zen of general practice

These days I work in some of the most poverty-stricken, chaotic, under-funded practices in the country. Places where you start 20 minutes late because they can't log you in, the printers don't go, the patients have scarily unwell bodies, no phones, no cars and they can't pay.

I love these patients and I love the people I work with, but I need to be Zen in the midst of the chaos and pressure. After a day flailing around in great waves of human need I feel wrecked, but not always, and it's the days when I finish energised that interest me. Apparently about 10 per cent of doctors finish their workdays with their tails wagging and their spirits zinging, so I'm sure the other 90 per cent of us can learn how.[1]

Recently one of our lovely young GP trainees said, 'But, Lucy, I feel so drained after a consultation like that.' We teach these young GPs communication skills by doing consultations with actors. In the role play he had just done, the patient wanted sleeping pills for stress, was in denial about early dementia, had been making mistakes at work, and her relationship was in tatters. The doctor was supposed to notice that her blood pressure was a bit high and discuss that with her in an understandable and inclusive manner. I gave them 40 minutes to get through it. I'm a realist.

But I'm also the teacher so I'm supposed to have wise things to say about how to stay sane despite the insanity of our jobs. Apparently, I've learned something from being burnt out. Maybe if I number my points and preach like a Facebook blogger, I will sound as if I know what I'm talking about. So, here's my listicle on finding the Zen of general practice:

1/ Treat yourself with care.

Apparently if doctors look after their work–life balance, do exercise and practise mindfulness, all will be well. This sounds easy but young doctors are often berated by their older colleagues for saying no, looking after themselves instead of sucking it up. Other times they are simply fobbed off as the *me generation.* Most of those doing the berating are men from what I call the *wife generation*, where the whole ethos of doctoring, the full-time-always-on-call-100-babies-delivered-a-year type of GP, depended on the support of a 1950s-style wife at home. Possibly I shouldn't fall into the trap of generalising another generation, but I do think the hardest thing in my medical career has been the lack of a wife. Without wife-care you need to do self-care. Or maybe just get a PA.

2/ Doing nothing can be doing something.

Quite often the most important thing I do is *listening.* Really. Listening is the thing. Listening is the doing. And I mean just listening: not listening while planning dinner, or listening while working out the next question I want to ask, or listening while waiting for a pause so I can take the blood pressure, or nodding-away sort of listening while wishing they would be quiet so I can do some real medicine. I mean when I put that all down, all of it, still myself and hear what is being said. People know when someone is listening in this way. And funnily enough the medicine gets done and often makes more sense, and that diagnosis or prescription or investigation we are so keen to get on with fits much more easily into the patient's story if we have listened first.

3/ There is enough time, even if there isn't.

When I am 40 minutes behind and the next patient bursts into tears and my mind goes, 'Oh no, heaven help me', I try to remember to breathe and say, 'There is enough time.' There is always enough time. And if I'm really stressed I place my feet on the floor and breathe again and feel my outbreath push that overwhelm down my legs, out through my shoes, into the earth. While still listening and not panicking about the people waiting. (A note for medical students studying anatomy: the breath does not, of course, literally go out the legs, but medicine is full of mystery and wonder and things that cannot be explained by dissection.)

4/ You can't fix everything.

Mostly we doctors want to fix things, do stuff to make it better. But the pain of life is seldom fixable, so perhaps there is only something to hear, a human being to see, one who is doing their best. There is mana to uplift, aroha to find, and in the end that might be more important than their cholesterol pills. At least for today.

5/ Discover calm.

Apparently if we are calm *outside* of work we will be able to find calm *inside* work when our computer suddenly freezes or the patient brings up life-threatening chest pain right at the end of their visit. I have achieved real calm a few times in my first 30 years of practice. It was incredible. I even had zing at the end of the day.

Don't get me wrong, for most of my career I have *looked* calm. I'm a doctor, I'm really good at looking calm. But it's not often *real* calm; it is a learned way we have of ignoring feelings and being disconnected from a body that is tense and agitated, all so that we can think clearly, which we need to do too.

I am realising that being truly calm is the sort of integration of my head, my limbs and my heart; an interconnectedness with people and things, past and present, which sounds awfully similar to what we teach in hauora Māori and makes me wonder who is teaching whom.

It's hard for doctors to integrate our own mind–body–soul complex because our Western medical model assumes the body is a machine and the mind is elsewhere. No wonder we struggle with maladies of the soul or just can't imagine our breath going out through our feet.

6/ 'It' is not mine.

The patient's problems are theirs. I know that sounds mean, so let me explain.

I like the idea that I am a witness, and when I witness there is a transaction that eases their burden or gives them the vigour to carry on. But I have to let that burden wash over me or through me or under me, because if I let it soak into me, I feel my own vigour drain.

It's important to acknowledge and empathise with the load being carried but we can only assist others if we are not weighted by 'it' ourselves. I think of myself as an observer sitting steady and calm in the swirl of it, noticing it, understanding it, offering suggestions and encouragement and yes, love, but I cannot carry it for them because I encounter so many 'it's in a day that if I try to carry them all, the sheer mass of it will crush me.

When I do feel the weight of it pushing on my shoulders, overwhelming me, I try to imagine lifting it up, shaping it into something smaller and lighter and giving it back to the patient, knowing and trusting they can carry it on their own.

7/ Unacknowledged feelings tend to spread around.

Sometimes for no apparent reason I can feel angry or tearful in the middle of a consultation and I realise that the person in front of me has unspoken feelings and I have absorbed them through some unconscious energy transfer, so I am now feeling the patient's feelings because maybe they are too hard for them to speak or know. I try to be curious about such feelings, not judge them, offer them back kindly, as possibilities.

These transfers of feeling can go from doctor to patient too, so the patient feels our unspoken feelings. I call this savage professionalism; the doctor who looks polite and benevolent but is actually projecting their own frustrations with the patient all over the room. Patients know when we are irritated with them even if we don't say it. They know when we are judging them. Can we acknowledge our own bad feelings to ourselves and allow them to drain out of our feet, lest they ooze out and infect the patient?

8/ Shake 'it' out.

My qigong master tells me to jump between consults. If you feel 'it' in your body, shake it out. While jumping and throwing my arms around I am to say this mantra: 'I'm getting rid of stagnant thoughts and feelings, and it will be OK.' This is definitely not in the medical school curriculum but it makes you feel so much better.

9/ Let them go.

My qigong man also claims he never thinks about a patient after they have left his consulting room. At first, I thought he was mad. I *have* to think about them. Isn't that reflective practice? Maybe. But maybe it's rumination, maybe it's being over-responsible, carrying the weight of something that is not mine to carry.

I wonder now if he is right. Perhaps the goal is to attend very closely to the person in front of me, then farewell them out the door and into their life, trusting that they have it in them to manage their troubles without me fretting.

10/ Laugh.

Recently a GP trainee sat in with me for an afternoon seeing patients. We found ourselves doing a lot of laughing. It felt unprofessional, a bit naughty, but we were not laughing at the patients, just the sheer absurdity of what we were trying to do in 15 minutes. Laughing really helped.

11/ Find some mates.

I know listicles always have only 10 things because all problems of living can be solved in 10 steps — not 5 or 12 or 1000, always 10 — it's kind of weird. In my listicle, number 11 is important: mates.

I don't want to call them colleagues or mentors or people who perform the rituals of professional supervision; we need all these people too. But we need mates: kindred spirits, those who understand our world of work, know the intensity of it, know how it stirs us and can laugh at the weirdness of it. Mates we can be honest with. We can't do this job alone.

I've nearly convinced myself with my own listicle. I sound like an expert. But I suspect most listicle writers, myself included, never actually do most of the things on their list. It's aspirational. We're only human.

4. Story

Story. A story is a sequence of events over time, often involving human characters. Stories are usually told about events that have already happened but sometimes there can be a wondering or prognostic surmising or hopeful reckoning about what might happen in the future story. Stories are typically told between human beings as a way of cementing relationship, revealing identity and making meaning out of events.

Putting burnout on my CV

I recently decided I will put 'Spectacular case of burnout' on my CV. In terms of reflective practice and professional development it has been a game changer. I have certainly learned a lot about how illness stories heal.

After the first few months I knew the only way forward was to be honest, especially within medicine. I had learned from patients that keeping secret stories is crippling. A year after my unravelling I gave a conference talk to around 500 people on the narrative identity of doctors and at the end I spoke briefly about my burnout. It seemed to be the only part of my talk people heard! I remember the huge number of colleagues who spoke to me afterwards, not about my talk but about their own stories: lonely stories of burnout, breakdowns, mental distress, hospitalisation.

I resolved the next year to tell my whole burnout story at the GP conference. It was a terrifying prospect, but I knew I was not alone.

To get myself to a place where I could tell that story, I first had to dismantle the shame. I booked in a cup of hot chocolate with my postgrad tutor, Hamish Wilson, who had written about shame in medicine. Shame, he pointed out, was a sense of not reaching some external but internalised standard of how to be a good doctor.

'So, what is that standard?' Hamish asked me with his usual

sparkly eye and raise of eyebrow.

'Oh, well, I'm a doctor, I can manage everything. I can work through lunch, do a day of energy-sapping consultations, then a night on call, manage tricky staff relationships, race home to feed the kids before the phone goes, respond to my deteriorating relationship with my partner and then go through a series of significant life events without flinching.'

'Mmm,' went the eyebrow.

'Oh, yeah, that's ridiculous,' I said. 'Why would I think doing all that was a good idea? That's a really dumb standard.'

It was a simple turning point. You can't be shamed by a standard you don't agree with.

My confidence had taken a massive hit, but I am pretty brave and I gave a talk that was viscerally honest. Many in the audience were wondering, struggling, thankful that someone had at last put words to it. Hamish was there, too, grinning away.

+

Burnout can make you feel 'other'. Burnout talks, webinars and papers are usually about 'other' doctors. Not us. Medicine has an elaborate set of rules for membership and a way of othering those who have drifted off the standard. Othering diminishes people.

Inevitably medical culture sees burnout as an individual problem. There has only recently been talk of unhealthy workplaces and how structural pressures where doctors cannot do their job well create a moral injury that leads to burnout.

You can almost hear the conversation at the medical school admissions committee. 'We need to try to filter out those vulnerable to burnout. They won't make it in medicine.'

For a while, I felt that there must be something about me that was not right; I had been doing medicine wrong. But now I can see that those characteristics that make me vulnerable to burnout also make me a very good doctor in particular situations: situations of complex, uncertain human dis-ease. We need all types of doctors, including my type.

Early on I read about burnout everywhere, desperate to understand what was happening to me. Much of the information was based on the Maslach Burnout Inventory. Created by Christina Maslach in the late 1970s, it defines burnout as a combination of emotional exhaustion, depersonalisation, an unfeeling response to people, a poor sense of professional accomplishment and using cynicism as a coping mechanism.

My burnout did not really feel like this, and I remember being slightly deflated that I did not fit the accepted definition. I don't think I was cynical or unfeeling towards patients and I felt I was still a good doctor — I was just mentally exhausted.

The Maslach inventory also focuses entirely on the individual and does not factor in the work context or anything happening in your life outside work, so if your child just died or your house got flooded, that doesn't count in your burnout score. Nor does a marriage break-up.

Maslach's definition of burnout is used so much it has become 'what burnout is'. This is an example of a collective folly of scientific research. The folly works like this: researchers who have never had burnout imagine what people who are really stressed at work might have in common and ask participants questions the researchers think will be important, then they create a 'definition' based on the bias of their original question selection. This methodology misses the nuances of lived experience because in science we do not value people's personal testimonies.

Maslach's scoring system also made me feel objectified, something medicine often does to patients. It was as if the relentless physiology of burnout, the shame, the loss of function and identity could all be neatly described with a few yes/no questions. It made me realise how disinterested medicine is in illness stories. Even now I feel like no one has really worked out what burnout is, and you can be left with the feeling you have nothing: it's all in your head.

In the beginning I was desperate to hear another story like mine, to know someone else had been through this. I needed to be told recovery was possible. That's why I decided to tell my story.

+

Part of the problem is medicine is more pressured than it used to be. Most GPs are drowning under so much stuff they can't look up to see the big picture. Funding is seriously constricted and there are more tasks, more inboxes, more health needs, more demands for reporting, more new treatments, more well-informed patients, more standards to meet. We could work day and night and never get it all done.

We may be drowning, but in medicine we have to keep going; that is one of the non-negotiable rules of membership. So we get thrown a life jacket and some flippers. Most of us say, 'I'm fine, give that to the poor doctor next door who really needs it.' The flippers offered by the burnout-prevention, building-resilience agencies end up in the back of the store cupboard behind the expired adrenalin and the bird flu-ready kit. However, studies show that most GPs have signs of impending burnout. Most of us are in the torrent.

If you are in this state, whatever your job, please do something radical. If you can, take six months off. Stop right now. Get out of the river you are drowning in, climb the bank, dry yourself off and lie in the sun. Stop. Look. Listen to your body. Everything will seem different, and you will know what you need. Stop.

Your workplace will survive without you. Your career will not end, the sun will rise tomorrow, and you will be different. Better, even. Stop. Your kids will suddenly be more loveable. You may not be given 'get well soon' cards or flowers or casseroles but you will have your life.

You can stay in the torrent and try a dose of care of self, but that might not be enough because burnout is not purely the absence of self-care. Of course, self-care helps but we also need to understand what the culture of medicine has done to us.

I still go to medical meetings where we talk about work stress, yet none of us leaves the windowless room all day. We talk at these meetings about self-care as the solution, and we think of it as an individual and private occupation, the benefit of self-care being apparent in a happy disposition, but the process of getting there invisible.

GP clinics can be really unhealthy places to work. There is an intense throughput pressure: more patients, more income. Tea breaks get put into the appointment diary but are seldom taken. Prior to Covid, very few practices had a process for covering a doctor who was sick, as if to say, 'Doctors can't get sick, because if they do, that just places stress on the rest of the team, so they better come back to work quickly.'

Our workload problem can be solved. Many things at a practice level could be done to reduce stress on doctors, but which doctor is going to put their hand up and say, 'Yes, we need to do things to care for us.' Doctors don't ask that; they do the caring. Until they can't.

+

So, what are protective factors against burnout? I suspect one factor is either a loving relationship in which you are supported and thriving, or being single. Chronically poor long-term relationships drain the life out of us. We are already 10 steps back when we walk in the door. (I might add that I do love my ex-partner. He's a fine fellow with a big heart, but we were not good at packing a car together.) Good workplace relationships are also hugely protective.

I would say that most people, GPs included, want to do *meaningful* work, but many structures and systems stop us doing the work that is important to us. Productivity is much easier to measure than meaning. Although, ironically, meaning generates productivity.

Fun can help. Laughing has a similar physiology to crying; it releases something from the body. Fun and medicine seem to be mutually exclusive. Medicine is a serious business, full of ethics and boundaries and professional behaviours. In that world, fun is a little risqué, but it is a great antidote to pressure.

A few years ago, I did a tour around the country, talking about fun and meaning as antidotes to burnout.

'How do you cope?' I said to a lovely fellow nearing retirement.

'I sing,' he said. 'And my colleague down the corridor sings too, so sometimes we sit in our rooms doing our paperwork and singing to each other.'

One GP I met was an expert at the mini kip. He would lock his door, lie on the examination bed with a blankie, shut the curtains, kip for just 10 minutes, and wake up refreshed.

I also spoke to GPs who prayed five times a day. Imagine if we all just stopped, knelt and wondered, even for five minutes, at something more meaningful than our tick-box performance scores? Perhaps, I thought, I could reclaim the rosary: a Hail Mary between patients and a Glory Be at the end of the day.

I have tried mindfulness, just being in the now, dealing with only the task in front of me, ignoring the huge pile lurking, and

I have to say it worked quite well — everything got done, no one died. It's a hard skill to learn, though.

Often I relapse to minimal self-care, pausing for a microsecond between patients, speed writing the notes then dashing out to collect the next patient, smiling graciously at my staff and stifling an internal frenzy of 'Shit, I'm running late'.

I am discovering that GPs have secret rituals used between patients. One young fellow does 20 press-ups after a particularly demanding consult. Another does a one-minute Headspace meditation, and one puts on his headphones after a challenging consultation, shuts the door and dances: 'It is great.'

One GP reported putting her hand on the closed door and saying, 'Go well', transferring the psychic energy she had just imbibed back to the patient or the universe. It works.

Between patients and behind closed doors, some GPs hold crystals. Another pops on a red spongy clown nose and laughs at herself in the mirror. One old fellow told me that once the patient is gone, he sticks his thumbs in his ears, waggles his fingers and pokes his tongue out.

What about the lovely one who strips down to his undies at the end of the day and does a 30-minute exercise routine before going home. He assured me that no one would catch him in his undies as he is always the last to leave. Of course. But I suggested his wife buy him some activewear for Christmas, just in case.

I have a friend, a magnificent GP, who is calm, considered and curious about his patients. I wondered how he maintained this approach.

'For the last twenty years I have meditated every morning,' he told me. 'I think I have spent so much time in that calm state, I notice as soon as something stresses me, and I can access calm again in one breath.'

Magic. Why didn't they teach me that in medical school? Doctors don't talk about such things.

What interests me now is what happens in the consultation that drains our energy. My friend is right. It's all in the breath. I have learned to listen to my body. It tells me there is a problem long before my mind realises. I have learned the power of staying calm in the face of all the stuff coming at me, the complexity, the feelings, including my own, the tension and pressure. I have learned that making a difference can only happen when I am well.

Mr Lucky

Yesterday, as I lay head down, feet up, ankles locked, on a contraption somewhat like a medieval torture table, I thought, 'I wonder what my doctor mates would think of this?' I was at my weekly treatment with Mr Lucky, my qigong master. I had gone to him because I was looking for a story for my weary aching body and was wondering if I might have a blocked chi, although I'm not sure what that is. I'm coming out of my burnout and fatigue still hampers me.

If I had gone to a rheumatologist, I might have got a diagnosis of fibromyalgia — I am tense all over with hyperalert trigger points. A rheumatologist might have given me some awful pain-relieving drug like amitriptyline and I didn't want that. And I was already yoga-ing, exercising, therapising and physio-ing.

So here I am, strapped into a medieval torture contraption, being tipped upside down by a smiling Mr Lucky.

I have become one of 'those' patients with an ill-defined malady for which medicine has no good answer. It's a revelation. Patients like me can make doctors feel awkward; they might even call me a 'heart sink' patient. Luckily, my marvellous GP has an appreciation of the mystery of life and the limitations of her prescription pad.

I told her all about Mr Lucky. The upside-down treatment is to help the flow of fluid around my body. The fluid has no anatomical or physiological substance or any resemblance to anything I learned in medical school. But the real challenge is to relax my legs, trusting that the ankle bracket will stop me sliding down onto my head. 'Let go,' says Mr Lucky, happily slapping my leg. 'Let go.'

Next is the pick-up-from-behind, in which Mr Lucky, who is very short, stands on a platform and plucks me off the floor in one swift lift. I go from fearing he might break me to telling myself, 'It's OK, he knows what he is doing, he's a quigong professional.'

'Accept,' he grins. 'Your chi is blocked in your chest.'

Really? Apparently, we doctors are slow learners. He's seen a few of us. Blocked chi feels right. I didn't learn about 'stories stuck in bodies' at medical school but the more I see of mysterious ailments, the more it makes sense to me.

Chi or no chi, it's onto the massage table I go. I'm loath to call it massage because the pain inflicted on my triggered muscles is excruciating, reminiscent of giving birth to a 10-pound baby. It's so painful the only option is, indeed, to let go.

After the first treatment, I woke in the night without a sign of muscle ache, as if my body had gone silent. 'Crikey,' I thought, 'I have taken a placebo and it's working.' I'm not sure we could do an evidence-based outcome study of Mr Lucky's upside-down, chi-moving, laughter-filled, pain-of-life-accepting clinic. But I'm happy to be an anecdote. And apparently I am unblocking — what, I do not know — but I definitely have a profound sense of well-being and much less aching. Truly, it's working.

I have been telling other GPs about Mr Lucky. Just about everyone has volunteered some fringe treatment that was helpful to them. Never mind evidence. More like whispered confessions: crystals, acupuncture, St John's wort, echinacea, hypnosis, Chinese medicine, laughter yoga, any old self-proclaimed chi shifter. Really, doctors are doing this. Who would have thought?

Back to Mr Lucky I go. May my chi be unstuck and my fluid flow freely.

On not being Ashley

It's 5 April 2020. The country is in lockdown. Waiting. The pandemic hasn't quite reached our shores but I feel a need to rise to the occasion, offer my services at the front line instead of faffing around as I have been, writing a book about being a doctor while doing little of it, and teaching others how to do it while wondering if I still have that sharpness in me, that quick pattern recognition, that diagnostic edge, that confidence that I know what I don't know, drug doses at my fingertips, that glorious feeling that I can do all of this and simultaneously manage the unexpected, the macabre, the lost and the uncertain.

I had imagined myself as a pandemic doctor giving unction to the dying in virus-infested houses in the poorer suburbs of the city where I now live, but in reality I have spent the week at my kitchen table doing telephone consultations in my socks.

I want to be heroic, as doctors are meant to be, but actually I'm terrified at the idea of exposing myself to a lethal load of virus while tending to those coughing, hoicking, drooling victims. Me, with no mask and no drugs. I have read the gruelling stories of doctors in Italy and New York. But this is New Zealand, and already some good keen bloke is in his shed making plastic face shields with his 3D printer and attaching these to small helmets and delivering them free to doctors around the country. I have one and I feel safer.

I love my country, a small string of islands in the south-west Pacific. I love blokes in sheds. I love that we have a female prime minister who is simultaneously toilet training her toddler and fending off a pandemic of catastrophic proportions. Every day I tune in at 1 p.m. for the Ashley Bloomfield Show, the weeks-old reality TV slot starring the nation's director-general of health. Today, Ashley tells us, we have 89 new cases. If it were 89 and a half, we know we can rely on Ashley to tell us and to explain the half.

We love him. He is the best of doctors. Calm and unruffled in a crisis, he spreads orderliness over the dizzying influx of numbers and graphs. There is no arrogance or condescension in him, none of the worst of medicine. He is kind. He's prepared to be wrong but seldom is because his world is not black and white; we are in an evolving situation.

He looks tired, as we would expect a doctor to look in a pandemic, and a national cheer goes up when we are told he is to have a day off. But he doesn't let himself slip. He wears a suit at every appearance and we can be sure he has washed his hands meticulously.

We trust him. We know Ashley Bloomfield couldn't tell a lie to save himself. The worst he might do is save some critical information for tomorrow's show, so that he has more of a handle on its implications.

I'd like to be the Ashley Bloomfield kind of doctor but I'm not. I've got bits of Ashley in me but I have a different job from him. I'm not sure how he would go delivering flu vaccines and good cheer in overheated council flats that smell of mutton fat and urine.

That was my job yesterday. I found a man alone and moribund, his grey blanket covered in blodges of tenacious phlegm. He wanted me to fix his headphones because his lifeline had been severed and he needed to be reinjected with talkback radio. He didn't want a flu vaccine and I suspect he was right; we were a bit late for prevention. He didn't want to go to hospital but in the end he went, and three days later he died alone. I just hope they got his radio going.

Next I visited a woman who couldn't get a ride to have her flu vaccine and she also needed her blood pressure checked because she had been started on more pills to bring it down. But the truth was she had not taken the new pills so her blood pressure was still high and then there was the problem of a repeat prescription for her large doses of morphine, which made me uncomfortable because we know she has a creepy son with a criminal history who may well be selling the morphine or using it himself in some sort of familial contra deal. I think she knew I would leave quickly when she mentioned that her son, *that* son, was about to call by.

+

Ashley is great but my situation requires another sort of doctor. I'm not sure I can explain without another story.

I confess I often call my patients *love* or *lovely*, as I do my friends and students and sometimes my colleagues (though probably not Ashley). I feel I need to explain myself. I like *lovely*'s softness. You can't say it unless you mean it. Sometimes it's different and I call them *sir* or *mate*, but seldom *dear*, although they are all dear to me in one way or another, even the man chucking grump down the phone at me, holding me responsible for his prescription problems when I know he had the sound off on his cell phone yesterday — I'd tried calling him four times — and didn't he know that overnight the nation's GPs had converted to 80 per cent phone consultations so people like him wouldn't have to sit in waiting rooms spraying viruses across the shabby spaces between plastic chairs? Didn't he think we docs were great the way we'd done that, like magic? Couldn't he have just obliged and had the sound up on his phone?

And no, I'm not interested in his plans to complain to the government about something I missed because I was momentarily distracted by thinking about the strangeness of telephone consultations and how he is in a supermarket picking up smokes and frozen pies while I'm in my kitchen looking at the grotty tiled floor hoping a cleaner will be allowed to come soon and remembering the washing needs to be hung, all the while trying to divert him from his rant to the topic at hand — his script — which he declares is urgent even though he hasn't needed it for the past nine months. I notice my teeth squeeze together as he has one more go at nasty and I get an unfamiliar feeling of real irritation with a patient. It doesn't happen to me often but we are both under a pandemic cloud and there is a squeezing tension in all of us.

By the end of the day, the grump and I are friends. He did get his overdue chest X-ray, as is always needed six weeks after someone has had pneumonia. It has been three months, and he tells me he can't breathe getting up to the house. I declined to give him controlled drugs for his pain of life in view of his history of addictions, even though he corrected me about his alcoholism, claiming that he now doesn't drink before lunch. I rang him back that evening, moments after I'd poured myself a soothing chardonnay in an elegant glass with a slice of washed-rind cheese on a gluten-free cracker, because the radiologist had found my phone number and told me the man's left chest was full of fluid.

Part of me wanted to finish that chardonnay and ring him in the morning, but I knew it was bad, so I tapped into my inner Ashley Bloomfield and picked up the phone. He was both scared and feisty, but we managed a laugh before he packed his bag and finished his fourth litre of scrumpy for the day and went off to hospital. I even heard his tail wagging.

I don't like hospitals. Those strutting young doctors, that

flurrying rush of nurses, those steely professors who know by the cut of me that I can no longer recite the verses of the Krebs cycle and have forgotten how to calculate a creatinine clearance. I confess I rely a little too much on Google. I know I can look those things up if I need to across town in my community clinic with its carpet worn down by the split soles of homeless people.

So, it's hard for me to send someone to hospital with their tail wagging but I seem to be able to do it. I don't know how. You have to position yourself as someone who can be trusted, but not in an arrogant way, more in a way that can share bad news lightly and cares enough to bother with at least one practical detail, such as how he will get there, given what we both know but don't say: that he is well over the limit and shouldn't drive.

It's hard work, even in person, to convince a frightened and surly stranger to understand the gravity of their situation and that they need to get to hospital. By phone it's even harder. I'm watching myself do this, listening to the tiny silences on the dark screen of my phone, hearing his hesitation, feeling my way, adjusting the plan, presenting it differently, talking it up while appearing benign, cheerleading him into doing what is medically prudent by harnessing the mate within, oversharing my own experiences, laughing at myself, telling him that 'the specialist agreed if you were our dad we would want you in hospital tonight'.

+

That was the moment he softened, this man I have never seen in the flesh, have only spoken to three times in one day by phone, but who I imagine is a little unkempt and lives in one of those houses in a flood-prone suburb; a house with a warm kitchen and a dreary hall and a shower with rising damp. But, all the same, I imagine he might have looked in the mirror and done his hair before picking up his bag, a comb-over type of look, and the bag a well-used giveaway from the Super Liquor store, and maybe it holds pyjamas from the back of his cupboard from a more dignified stage of his life, but probably it is my wishful thinking that there had been such a time and he in fact packed an old T-shirt and what my nephew calls fat pants.

I imagine he might have felt good: a man with a bag in a taxi with his hair slicked down. But then I worry that he might have felt small as he was delivered to the emergency department, because during our second call he had told me with rising agitation how his father had whipped him with a belt every day and sometimes he had cried and then he had been beaten more. He had PTSD, didn't I know? And I told him I'd read something about that in the notes. It had been on the list after emphysema and dyspepsia and fractured metacarpals and hepatitis C — but I had felt it in him anyway, and so later on I hoped he wasn't gruff when he walked into the emergency department, because the health system, too, can give a whipping to those who are unkempt or ungracious or wounded, even if they have combed their hair.

And I called him *lovely*, and I said I would ring him next week to see how he is doing, and I will.

Story of a pain

Last year I had a strange experience. I was walking a muddy hiking track and I'm pretty sure I took a big step down, did an uneasy pivot on my right leg and strained my groin. I took some ibuprofen and carried on. It was a slight niggle, but a week later walking down a hill the pain reappeared, worse than ever.

The story of this symptom didn't quite make sense in my doctor mind, and I've seen enough patients to know that the mind and body don't act independently, so I asked myself, 'What is my body trying to tell me?'

Life was pretty good so I went back to a physical cause for the pain. I did a self-examination, as doctors do, but it was hard to work out what the problem was. I thought about the medical possibilities: osteoarthritis of the hip (OA), a tendon strain or maybe a labral tear. I went home and Googled labral tear of the hip cartilage and that turned out to be a bad idea because it can be tricky to treat. I didn't want it to be one of those.

I was starting to worry. If I had OA I might have to stop walking either for a few weeks or, God forbid, a long time. Walking is my sanity so that wasn't a good thought. And I don't have medical insurance, so I'd have to dip into retirement savings to get a hip replacement.

I was getting well ahead of myself, so I told myself to calm down. After all, odd pains often just go away. I kept walking, adding in a few stretches and some more ibuprofen. The pain got worse.

I have a great GP. By the time I saw him I was a few weeks into the thing, and I was taking paracetamol and ibuprofen four times daily. I could do short walks on the flat but couldn't sit for long periods. I saw him on Wednesday, had a hip X-ray on Thursday, with a normal result on Friday. It was a relief I didn't have osteoarthritis. I had an appointment for physio the next Monday and a referral to a specialist in case we needed to rule out that labral tear.

But on the Friday night I had terrible pain. I had to take codeine to sleep. Luckily there was some left in the cupboard from my son's orthopaedic surgery. I know doctors are not supposed to self-treat, but let's face it, bathroom cupboards around the country are a rich source of leftover medications that people try even when they ought to know better.

I have to confess I woke a bit concerned. Muscle and tendon strains are normally worst at the beginning and gradually improve, so the pattern wasn't quite right. It was Saturday so I couldn't talk to my GP. 'I've probably just given it another tweak,' I thought.

On Saturday night the pain was worse and I needed two doses of codeine. By Sunday morning I was limping and had intense pain if I sat in a chair for more than 15 minutes. My mind was desperately trying to make sense of what was going on: 'Maybe I have something weird, what about a tumour deep in my right pelvis? Mmm, yeah, that could be it. I could be a goner.' The rational part of my doctor brain could not quell the fear.

I told my partner we were going to the emergency department, that I needed to be checked out. But just at that moment my old mate, who is also a GP, popped around to borrow a garden tool. He raised an eyebrow when I said I was going to ED, took a history and suggested he have a look at me. I know doctors are not supposed to look after friends, but I trusted him.

He said he didn't think a pelvic tumour was high on the list. He suggested better pain relief, crutches and rest. We could review the situation in a few hours. The pelvic tumour still lingered in my mind, but I felt slightly reassured by his pragmatism. Having a plan helped. Common things happen commonly, and maybe the pain would settle if I stopped walking around on it. It was a relief to believe him; I could just relax and stop monitoring the symptom.

He arrived back with a set of crutches from his neighbour's garage and told me to take more of my bathroom cupboard codeine plus 1600 milligrams of Brufen SR from my tramping first aid kit and some omeprazole to protect my tummy. My partner and my friend tucked me into bed, propping my leg up with pillows. I woke two hours later completely pain free for the first time in weeks. Wow, I thought, how weird. The pain never came back. Really. Never. One minute I thought I had cancer. Next minute: pain gone.

I've asked myself how on earth that had happened. Was it just that I trusted my friend, felt reassured and got tucked into bed? Or was it that I believed the story he gave me? Maybe the 1600 milligrams of ibuprofen had a massive peak drug level that switched off the pain and stopped the cycle of pain, worry, more pain, more worry.

I'm a rational doctor so surely it wasn't placebo! My friend had said the Brufen SR would work much better than the same dose spread over the day. He may even have said, 'It's magic stuff.' Maybe I believed him.

(Those Brufen SR are now my favourite prescription for anyone in pain. We doctors call it evidenced-based decision making.)

Story doctor

I often think that a medical consultation is an awkward collision between science and story. The patient brings a story of their unwell body but also a story of their life. Doctors bring medical science, which is pretty good at fixing bodies, but often we are faced with stories that need healing.

Consultations privilege the medical version of the story. When a patient tells a doctor about their illness, the doctor responds in a ritualised way, translating the story into a medical language inaccessible to the patient. If the patient is lucky, the doctor translates the story back again in order to explain the diagnosis and treatment.

Doctors record these stories in a coded form in medical records and in communications between health professionals. Depending on who tells the medical story and for whom, elements of the story are emphasised or excluded.

Frequently the patients lose their identity in the medical story, so when I tell you this is a story about Patient X, doctors will immediately understand what type of story they are going to hear. Patient X's story was first told to me as a simple sequence of events on an accident compensation form: 'Female, 34, fell off a retaining wall hurting back, 11 p.m., three weeks ago, occupation, shop assistant.'

I had not met Patient X before. She had a weary face and a musty jacket and as I greeted her I sensed the feeling of her. This sensing of someone is not considered part of the medical story and is not included in the medical record.

Patient X told me a story about her body, and she had already rehearsed the particular version of that story to tell the doctor. Later when she meets her friend for a beer, her story may be told with different words, subplots, emphasis and tone.

Patient X was what doctors call a perfect historian, a history in medicine being the story of bodily symptoms. A history is something a doctor takes. A doctor would say Patient X required no interrogation, interrogation being a form of persistent questioning doctors do in order to extract the information they want from the patient in an orderly manner. Patient X did not need interrogation; she told me the mechanism of injury, the site of back pain, the analgesia taken, the stoical going to work. There were no red flags — red flags being particular word sequences that alert the doctor to the possibility of something serious.

I listened to Patient X's story with my doctor's ear, filtering out irrelevant information, comparing her story with other back pain stories, looking for patterns, and sensing whether there was anything not quite right about this symptom story. I examined her to find evidence to support my story that not much was wrong with her back, while also being open to the idea I might find something that would make me review my story.

I recorded the medical story in what is called a patient's chart, a chart being a document that records progress or plots a course. A medical chart is a story without frills or subjectivities: 'Fell R buttock, ongoing pain localised to L4 R, no neurology, IMP Non-specific lumbar back pain. Refer physio, analgesia as charted. Reassured. TCI if persists or leg pain.'

These skills of history taking, information filtering, pattern recognition and objective observation are critical in the diagnostic process. However they can become problematic when the patient brings a story that is not just of their body.

Patient X's consultation sounds pretty straightforward but the curious thing was that the whole time she spoke tears streamed down her face. There was no relationship between the tears and the story coming out of her mouth, as if I was witnessing two stories simultaneously.

Most of what happened between Patient X and me was not recorded in the chart: my internal response, the things unspoken, the quiet handing over of tissues, the ritual examination accompanied by weeping, the silence into which I spoke.

'What is it that makes you cry?'

I was expecting a significant plot twist, something else going on in her life. To my surprise she said, 'I gave up smoking yesterday.'

I felt relieved but time was running out, patients were queuing up, and I needed to do tasks to complete the medical story.

'Have you given smoking cessation advice? Yes/No,' demanded my computer.

I ticked the 'Yes' box, handed over more tissues and disclosed my own story of giving up smoking. Obviously that story did not go into the medical record.

When Patient X was gone, I was left with a mystery. Was she really crying because of stopping smoking? What was missing from this story? Had she been pushed from the wall? Was she a drinker? Had her back pain unleashed some previous trauma?

We can think of this back pain story as a small paragraph in a chapter from the long book of Patient X's life. I had extracted a small and particular story about her body, not knowing what had come before or even what else was happening in this chapter. It would be easy for my extract to have missed the point.

In these small stories called consultations, doctors can take or be given roles; doctors like to play a slightly grand part, but the story and the patient determine what role we shall have. We often feel we were the hero who discovered the diagnosis and had solutions ready, only to later find the patient cast us in a non-speaking role. Sometimes, we think we have simply listened and done nothing, only to hear it was life changing.

I think Patient X felt better as she left. She had stopped crying, she didn't feel so musty, she may have smiled. She accepted the prescriptions and referrals I handed her as if they were evidence she had been heard and that something in her story was going to change.

But I was left feeling I had missed something important in this story, that this had not been a very good consultation. How would I know? It is reassuring to remember my superb GP teacher, Pat Farry, who told me, 'Lucy, in thirty years of general practice I think I have only done three good consultations.'

I can only know how this consultation seemed through my eyes, which is always going to be a limited and particular view. Patient X would no doubt tell the story of this consultation differently and her perception might surprise me.

+

We can't really say what a good consultation is unless we ask what a consultation is for. What is the purpose of medicine? To diagnose and treat disease? To relieve suffering? To improve well-being?

How might I have alleviated Patient X's suffering? Reassurance the pain would end? Pain relief? Time off work? Offering tissues? A faint touch on her arm as she left the room? Perhaps I needed to ask one more question to hear an untold story. Perhaps a moment of kindness was sufficient.

Medicine has powerful tools for relieving suffering: diagnoses, drugs and surgery. But getting the medical part right is seldom enough because there is not a linear relationship between the medical treatment and the reduction in suffering.

At times the delivery of the medical story can be so emphatic, and so lacking in curiosity and compassion, that it can silence the patient's story or add to their suffering.

Sometimes there is a diagnosis but there's no treatment for their problem. When the medical story doesn't know how to write the next chapter, the patient can be left navigating the illness on their own.

Often people suffer but we cannot find disease in their bodies, so we have no drugs or surgery to fix them. When doctors can't create a medical story for the symptoms, we sometimes minimise them, imply it isn't too bad and thereby increase the suffering.

Patients usually create a story to make sense of their symptoms but sometimes they're not aware they have done this and don't reveal this story to the doctor. In any case doctors are trained to filter out the patient's ideas and concerns. However when we ignore the patient's version, we leave their concerns unanswered, causing confusion and more suffering.

Sometimes the bodily symptom was unconsciously an acceptable way to bring their struggling life to the doctor, so the medical story misses the point. We also know people can be successfully diagnosed and medically treated but mysteriously their suffering continues.

+

When I was a house surgeon in a provincial hospital, I assisted a surgeon to remove an abdominal tumour the size of a football. It took us four hours to meticulously dissect it out, and it was so pleasing to throw it into a steel bucket and send it for histological testing. I remember the feeling of looking after that woman post-op and how well we did, her great recovery and, the icing on the cake, no cancer. A happy ending and a medical job well done.

Two years later I met that woman's son in the street and he remembered me. I asked after her, and he told me a story I will never forget.

'She's OK now,' he said, 'but she was very ill for a long time after that surgery, stayed home, couldn't work, the GP couldn't find anything wrong. But it's OK. We took her home, she's seen the tohunga and she's all good. Māori sickness.'

+

If we think in terms of disease that resides in the body and illness that resides in a person's life story, then suffering needs both a medical doctor for the disease and a story doctor for the illness.

In medicine we talk about patients as diabetics or asthmatics or borderlines, assuming all people with these diagnoses are the same. But each person with a disease also has a unique life story and a particular response to the diagnosis we have given them.

As story doctors we need to understand story sovereignty. I know I have a biomedical coloniser in me, a paternalistic part that wants the patient to take my medical story and use it to make their life better. In this narrative imperialism, the biomedical story can colonise the patient's story, and in that moment the patient's sovereignty begins to disappear. I can hear myself with my patient with diabetes, telling them the medical story in multiple different ways, urging them to see the truth of it and to comply with my advice.

But the patient needs to decide what will make their life better. They might need time to consider my medical story, decide whether they buy it and work out how to integrate it with their story. Sometimes this results in rejecting or denying the medical story. Perhaps it is our job to remain steady, kind and curious in the face of these deliberations.

My biomedical coloniser might have seen Patient X's tears and given her a sheet of Yes/No questions and counted those yeses and given her a symptom score and proclaimed, 'My big bible of psychiatric diagnoses is full of tidy little taxonomies, and you fit in the box called depression.'

Perhaps that would have helped her move her story to a better place. A diagnosis might have affirmed her experience and made her feel she was not alone, the prescription for Prozac a symbol of hope. I might have felt I had done something.

Or that diagnosis might have harmed her, made her feel she was deficient in some way. The label might have felt like a strange side plot imposed on her story by someone else.

I think at best this might have given Patient X a temporary narrative, one that she is free to accept or reject at any time. In the end, even if we think patients have depression, or psychosis or a borderline personality, they all have stories separate from those diagnoses. The patient needs to reclaim sovereignty over their story, create their own meaning and their own future life.

+

Illness impacts a patient's story, so to be story doctors we need to understand the characteristics of stories. Stories are how we make sense of things and each other. When we tell a story, we tell who we are, what is important to us, and we attribute meanings to happenings. Stories are dynamic because the telling of a story changes the teller's relationship with it, so the story alters the next time they speak it.

We edit a story, tell it slightly differently or leave bits out depending on who is listening because we are hoping to elicit a positive response, and we know that listeners have their own values, biases and judgements. We constantly assess which parts of our story are safe to share.

We tend to retell our stories in a way that portrays us in the best possible light, so the same sequence of events can create very different narratives. A man who punches his wife might tell me she started it. She will say she lives in terror. Another woman will tell me for years about her troubles at work, her worries about her kids and her husband's indifference to her. Later, after her death in a car accident, he will tell me she was an alcoholic.

Stories are a series of events over time. Doctors like medical stories in a temporal sequence but annoyingly patients seldom tell stories beginning to end. We call these people 'poor historians' because their storytelling does not fit our model. The doctor likes to know when and how the symptom started but the patient may be vague on this because it is only when a symptom impacts on their story that it becomes important to them.

Patients often bring a list of stories. The doctor's heart sinks because they like one story at a time. Inevitably the last story (often about fifth on the list and already 25 minutes in) is the most important, the most frightening, the most difficult to tell.

Sometimes it feels as if the first story is a test to see whether we can be trusted with the next story. Recently I saw a stranger who told me a long tale of his diabetes, high blood pressure and medications. Ten minutes in I asked, 'So do you need a prescription or a blood test?'

'No, I've had bloods and I have plenty of pills.'

Baffled, I asked, 'So what is your question?'

'Well. Um. I can't get a hard-on.'

Story sovereignty and the process of storytelling, listening, meaning making, retelling and editing are integral to understanding how to be a story doctor.

+

How can a story doctor help people with their injured stories? How can future stories start to be imagined? When I was a young GP, a complete stranger walked into my room, sat down and wept. Tissues being my most important prop, I handed them over silently. In fact, for the next 40 minutes I barely spoke. To my amazement the woman told me the story of her husband's affair, gathered her own coherence, recognised her own resources and decided what she needed to do. I felt I had done nothing.

What I have learned is that stories need listeners. Listening can take time, but the 40 minutes we invest in the first interaction lays the foundation for the next 2 or 10 or 20 consultations. Stories need to be told, for it is in the telling of our story that we also hear and start to understand it ourselves. We can tell stories to an internal audience in our head but there is something about storytelling that is relational.

Illness stories need safe listeners because illness poses a threat to a patient's personhood, a threat to their future imaginings of themselves, an interrupted narrative.[1] When we, as doctors, ourselves become patients, when we try to speak our illness story to another doctor, we come to understand how fearful illness is: fear of disease, fear of judgement, fear of looking stupid, fear of being misunderstood, fear of shame and, ultimately, fear of death.

Sometimes we sense the patient has an unspoken story. I may not have heard Patient X's full story, but I hope that I conveyed without words that I had heard something.

Many illness narratives cannot yet be spoken in words. Some stories remain untold for a reason. Stories of trauma come packaged with judgement, shame, fear of exposure and the need to protect others. Sometimes incoherent, they are very difficult narratives to tell. Horrific stories. Testimonies of such dimensions that we want to retreat.

Wordless stories can be told by the body, perhaps in metaphors: 'I can't swallow', 'My chest hurts', 'I can't stomach it', 'I have a pain in the neck'. Medical science sees the mind and body as separate so we cannot acknowledge that which the body speaks. Medicine calls these symptoms functional, a psychosocial problem, a moral weakness.

Complex trauma stories can come out slowly, in symbolic ways, or they are told indirectly, with inexplicable, often unappealing behaviours and complex re-enactments in which the doctor is unknowingly cast in unwanted roles. These patients baffle us, challenge, upset us, but it all starts to make sense when the story becomes known.

What stories seem to require is a witness. According to the psychologist Kathy Weingarten, a witness is someone prepared to grasp 'even for a second the experience of another'.[2] Witnesses need to be brave and unshockable, suspending judgement.

The story may call out for diagnosis, drugs or surgery but no matter how straightforwardly *medical* the story seems, there is something to witness, an experience of another to grasp. Witnessing is that moment where we let go of our doctor selves, the moment when we become very still, quiet.

When we have witnessed a story without judgement, shame or horror, the patient can potentially do this for themselves. To become the compassionate observer of one's own story is to become its future author.

The witness has to position themselves internally so that they truly suspend judgement. The patient will sense our judgement even if we do not speak it. We also need to learn to love those who seem unlovable because, as Professor Ian McWhinney, the grandfather of general practice, concludes: 'In the end . . . we are healed by love.'[3]

Sometimes we are just given fragments of the story. We are compelled to imaginatively fill in the gaps. We want to respond to the suffering, to act, do or say something to make it better. But first, pause. We need to build some sort of space to hold this story. It is hard for me to put this space into words, but I will try.

When we become still, we feel the story hovering between the teller and the witness in what writer Gillie Bolton calls the liminal space: the threshold between the rooms each inhabits.[4] Sometimes the story looms over the liminal space as a vague cloud, sometimes as a menace, but always it requires us to look because something important is before us.

The witness who has been prepared to open the door, to look into the liminal space, is handed a precious gift: a story. What happens next is a mysterious transaction between teller and witness.

We feel the weight of responsibility for it. Our cognitive minds kick back in to rescue us. Medical imperialism drives us to impose a plot, to know what to do, have a plan. Doctors are programmed to fix things. I think we do best with these stories when we hold a position of 'not knowing', accepting the mystery with curiosity, seeing that it is not ours to fix, that it may not be fixable in any way we understand.

'Not knowing' means sitting at the edge of the threshold with a person, quiet and still, for just a little longer. For in that stillness we accompany without words, we listen with a part of ourselves beyond language and thought. We listen to and with our bodies.

Words come and something tells us when the time is right to

speak. Words too soon can shut the door. Sometimes part of us wants to shut it, to not see. But to shut that door is to leave the other alone with their suffering.

First we must acknowledge what we have heard. It sounds easy but it's all about the right words, tone, volume and pace. It's a positioning of our body, the timing of our breath, the trueness of our gaze. If we get it wrong the suffering story will need to be repeated until we can show we have heard.

We are trained as doctors to look at people through a lens of deficits but sometimes when I hear a particularly traumatic story, I think, 'How has this person survived? Why did they not just crawl into a corner and die?' And in that moment I know that they survived because of their strengths, however fragmentary they might appear. When we see the patient in this way, we place their capacities in the liminal space with their story. These capacities power future imaginings of self, how life might be, beyond the present crises. Deficits impede stories; strengths propel them forward.

And then there is hope. Sometimes the patient has generated their own hope through this process but often we, as witnesses, have to hold hope until the person can access it. This is a complex internal process because we cannot convey meaningful hope unless we really are hopeful, and some stories are relentlessly traumatic and overwhelming. Our job is to know there are future possibilities for any story.

We can offer ways forward, but these offerings are not advice and there is no requirement that our offerings will be accepted. Offerings are about suggesting possible future pictures, giving permission for paths to be chosen, creatively imagining different ways of being or things to try.

The more time we spend listening to patients, the more we learn how people navigate terrible things. If we let the patient with the lived experience become the expert, they will teach us what helps and how stories can be changed.

Doctors need to be patient. Some stories take years or decades to change and there is no quick fix. But we need to accompany, sit quietly in the chaos, and trust. Perhaps with these skills a medical doctor can become a story doctor.

+

And Patient X? We had a curious follow-up at the supermarket checkout, as you do in a small town. She wanted me to know her back was fine; she hadn't needed the pain relief or the physio. But she had finally left her boyfriend. I didn't even know she had a boyfriend, but she seemed to think she had told me.

'Great,' I said.

'Thanks so much,' she replied.

An apologetic defence of my longer consultations

I suppose the problem is that I didn't become a doctor to deliver HealthPathways. Don't get me wrong: I love them. They provide doctors with comprehensive guidelines on how to diagnose and treat all manner of diseases using all the latest scientific evidence. They are better than Google and thank goodness they exist because I have forgotten half of what I once knew.

But most of my patients have dis-eases that don't have a health pathway, or they have so many problems that I'm not sure which pathway to follow and whether it matters anyway because in the end they often come up with some random, unexpected reason for their dis-ease; not their blood pressure or diabetes at all but something else, that other thing, just expressed in a little pause at first, an odd word in a sentence that seems a bit lost or perhaps a shuffling attempt to make utterances at all.

The blood pressure and the diabetes are the easy bit. I just click and up comes the evidence-based pathway with everything I need to know: other diagnostic possibilities, tests to do, drugs to prescribe, pro formas for funded annual diabetic checks, health literacy improvement patient information sheets, chronic disease well-being and self-efficacy flow charts, personal care plans, acute care plans, advanced care plans and client-led comprehensive health assessments checklists — they are all there at the click of a button. I can even measure my outcomes. You would think with all that help I could get through the consultation in 15 minutes.

The problem is that I am addicted to following the cues. Recognising cues is a medical education communication skills advanced competency. It's probably best to think of them as clues: bits of the story that don't quite fit, the add-on at the end of a sentence easily glossed over, the particular description of someone else who wasn't obviously part of the story. Sometimes the clues are more like weathervanes, a sense of something brewing beyond the symptoms, but sometimes the clues are great big flashing beacons with sirens such as wordless weeping, rage, bottomless pain or evasive silence.

But I find that more and more I am compelled to follow them. The human pathway is so much more interesting than the health pathway. The patient leads and I follow. Well, they are not really leading because the patient isn't sure of the path either, so maybe I am just accompanying them, wondering about possibilities, pondering crossroads and perhaps suggesting we take a look down this one, even though I have no idea where it leads, and I ought to be more prudent because I am already 30 minutes behind, and people are waiting.

But I can't help myself. It feels disrespectful not to notice the clue, as if somehow the patient is expressing shyly that, really, they want to talk about *this* thing, rather than their blood-sugar testing, but when I say 'want' I don't mean consciously want in the sense that they planned to talk about that thing when they made their appointment. I don't think it often works like that. They were coming to talk about their blood sugar but something in the safety of the room, in the knowing that the doctor has heard such things before, can keep a secret and will be unshockable, means that *it* just slips out, unconsciously, into a sentence about something else.

Like the man who goes, 'Yes, I have had a sore throat and a cough and I've been pretty stressed, but I'm coughing up a bit of phlegm.' Spot the word that doesn't fit the sequence. Should I ignore the 'stressed' and just stick to my doctor things: the throat, the cough and the sputum? Don't I need to do both? And sometimes the stress isn't much of a thing, but the throat is, and other times the consult is all about the stress and the throat was just a legitimate way for a troubled fellow to get some help.

So yes, I should be able to discuss their blood sugars and throats and prostates and piles in 15 minutes but something always sabotages that, and I just can't pretend I didn't hear it, that faint whisper of some story other than the one we are on.

+

And sometimes it's not so subtle. Many of my patients nowadays exist in the substrata below the radar that counts people in our country. They may have blood-sugar ills but they never make it to specialist appointments or get X-rays or do blood tests. Taking their insulin is just not a priority in a life swamped in trauma and poverty and trying to keep clear of the cops. They are beautiful people, all of them, doing their best, helping their mates and fighting their demons, but there are times when I desperately want their blood sugars to be better and I start to lecture them on weight and exercise and a diet they can't afford, all for their own good. But then I feel my folly, shut myself up and tell them instead that they are marvellous, and their blood sugar can wait until they are feeling better; after all, it's been that high for years so probably another few weeks won't matter.

And then, just when I let it go, and realise the best I can do here is treat this person with respect, this woman who was abused in foster homes and raped by a man of the cloth and is still going, still going, still able to crack jokes, and smile and cry simultaneously, this woman who has never been treated with respect — yes, maybe my respect is the best thing I can give her — just in that moment when I thought that, before I had even said anything, she senses it in me and her tail starts to wag, a little minor beat at first, then still but somehow ready to wag again.

I always feel I have done a good job if the patient leaves with their tail wagging. An analogy that compares a patient to a dog is possibly disrespectful but I'd argue that the tail of the dog is the gold standard visual cue to the internal state. Some patients wag because they have a better script in their hand for a better pill to make their blood sugar even better; some wag because their diet and exercise programme has helped and the doctor has patted and patted them for their lovely notebook of blood sugar tests all in the same coloured pen; some people wag because they are just naturally waggers so why wouldn't you wag coming out of a doctor's office; and sometimes blokes wag if, for example, they've had some problems with their back passage, and they were able to say it and we have gone through the embarrassment of sorting it, so now we can relax and talk about not putting sugar in their tea.

But the patients who come with their tails between their legs, hunched in retreat or snarling through their teeth, they are the hard ones. It's a challenge to find their marvellousness but they are the ones to pat, not straight away, of course, just easing forward, being small and quiet, speaking little and slowly, edging closer, until perhaps that tail relaxes.

+

I'm sounding grandiose now, like a sort of benevolent patient whisperer. I'm not that good at all. And I'm a problem in a medical centre because doctors are income-generating units and the unit of time is 15 minutes, otherwise the accounting doesn't work.

I've been lucky; practice partners have seen the value of my approach and were prepared to pay me for my time rather than my measurable productivity, although no doubt they started to wonder what on earth I was doing in there. And I had moments of wondering myself: Could I do this faster, more efficiently, with less meandering? Once, for a few months, during my relationship break-up, I did. I recognised I wasn't in any place to listen to other people's troubles so I lost the desire to pick up cues. I was friendly and polite, I addressed the throats and prostates and piles, wrote scripts, gave information and ran on time.

I felt like a proper doctor, one of those straightforward colleagues who prides themselves on professional boundaries and up-to-date competencies; the ones who know that maladies of the soul are not their concern and appropriately refer these patients to a mental health service or health improvement practitioner or any type of specialist, like a cardiologist, rheumatologist, endocrinologist, gynaecologist, dermatologist, neurologist, pathologist or urologist, the choice being determined by which anatomical body part seems most afflicted.

Sometimes these referrals help and sometimes they don't because it takes a long time to be seen, and the waiting itself is harrowing, and sometimes the specialist has no answer because the body part they deal with is not anatomically linked to the soul that is aching, or the mental health team uses a diagnostic categorising app that gives a label, which can be reassuring but offers no hope or meaning to the patient.

+

I am supposed to teach GP trainees to pass a clinical exam which consists of 10 consultations with actors, 14 minutes each. They pass despite me. I am supposed to teach them communication skills models, and I do love some of the elements of these models, such as the idea of not interrupting the patient in the first seven seconds the way most doctors do, or the idea of safety netting or summarising or finding out the patient's expectations or — the most important one of all — finding out what the patient thought the problem was in the first place. Because if the 15-year-old thinks their rash is due to picking up a sexually transmitted disease from going to third base (mouth to genital) but the doctor doesn't even have sexually transmitted infection on their differentials and therefore doesn't get into the territory of third base, then the consultation will be unsatisfactory for the patient, their questions will be unanswered and they will be left to face the hazards of fourth base (genital to genital) alone.

I dislike the linear nature of consultation models, as if one step happens directly after another when, in fact, consultations are situations of chaos and complexity, like the fellow giving the clue 'trouble with the kids' in the middle of something unrelated while I am busy thinking about his symptoms and wondering if he could have had a blood clot and is it too late to send him to the lab today, and simultaneously, because blokes are seldom frequent flyers at the GP, the computer is flashing at me: he is overdue for checks for weight, height, BMI, BP, blood sugars, cholesterol and cardiovascular risk score, and why not update his tetanus and offer a flu vax and one for shingles and make sure he did his bowel screening. And just then I notice he is overdue for his PSA test, and in that moment, he says, 'Oh, and I've been pissing blood.'

I can't fathom how any model can make this linear, although I do accept part of my 15-minute task is extracting some order out of chaos, translating unspoken clues, rapid prioritisation, assessing risk, making plans, witnessing pain and suffering with compassion, problem-solving, logistics, considering fair distribution of resources and conveying reassurance in the face of uncertainty while simultaneously noticing the guy also has a tremor on one side, which is concerning but maybe not today's problem.

So yes, I find the linear model with a pathway of tick-box achievements that can measure the doctor's performance a little simplistic. Consultations are seldom linear. They are circuitous, they are juggling acts with multiple balls, they bounce around between certainty and uncertainty, they involve wireless transfers of energy and information and feelings and that which cannot be spoken and mysteries and magic.

Consultations are not always best when we doctors have our medical agenda and lead the way, unbidden, into our own list of things to accomplish. We need to know when to lead and when to follow, when to speak and when to be quiet, and when to just shut up and leave a pause for some other knowing to come from the patient who is, after all, the centre of the encounter, not us. It's not all about us. Us, with our tidy diagnoses and data to collect and things to administer and end goals to measure. No, sometimes we need to follow and follow and follow the patient some more until we have come around in circles to the point where we started but now understand something that needed knowing before we could move on to the medicine.

No, it's not all about us, but sometimes it is. Sometimes we are on a roll with our explanations and certainties, and sometimes that is just the right thing for the patient, but we can't assume it is. If we notice when we have been a bit too full of ourselves, and at the end of all our interrogating and categorising and explaining and referring and safety netting, we also notice that there is no tail wagging, somewhere in there, we have missed the point.

Coloniser tends those dispossessed by colonisation

It's tricky writing about being a Pākehā doctor to Māori. The coloniser tending to those dispossessed by colonisation is always an awkward dance. The doctor's room is itself a politicised venue, like entering an inner sanctum where we expect the patient to worship all that we stand for. We ask them to believe: in us, in what we think is best for them, in a Western version of health, which is essentially health for those privileged enough to not be worried about housing or work or putting food on the table or dealing with government agencies who will judge them.

Sometimes we sing from the missionary's hymnbook: 'Swallow my pills and you will be healed.' Sometimes we pull out our great bible of health literacy and translate it into simple language for those we assume know nothing of health at all.

Sometimes we go on a crusade, mount a drive-through of the poorer indigenous suburbs, dropping health pamphlets from our high horses.

Sometimes we say it is their fault if they die young; we can't be responsible for poor life choices like chicken nuggets and Coke, while those in power have imported blue cheese with sips of Perrier because French water must be better.

Sometimes we get millions of dollars to research the problem and we peer at *them* through our telescopes, then build careers on our pompous conclusions, claiming we are the ones who know why these people have poor health outcomes.

It works on paper, that mission to drive down the rate of diabetes and kidney transplant and alcohol abuse. It makes absolute sense in terms of epidemiology and equity and public health and fairness, written neatly in a manifesto in an office, downtown, where the dispossessed are kept out by security guards.

+

It's much harder when I am face to face with real people like Aroha. Aroha hasn't been to a doctor for 30 years and confesses to having a beer in the car before her 10 a.m. appointment. She only came because she needed a letter for Kāinga Ora Housing New Zealand, or maybe it was Te Hiranga Tangata Work and Income, or perhaps it was for Oranga Tamariki, who have control over her moko, or possibly some other agent of state that is requiring my assessment and approval before they will offer her any concessions.

My sense of Aroha is she is wounded. But she is also ātaahua, brave and honest, doing her best to move her whānau out of the wilderness of the dispossessed into some other place. She wants somewhere for her whānau to put their feet. She also wants me to pronounce Kāinga Ora properly. For some reason, not quite clear to me, we do a lot of laughing.

She refuses my blood test to screen her for diseases that run rife in the Māori population but she does have a cervical smear, her first ever. I'm not sure I could explain why she suddenly agreed to me placing a speculum in her vagina when all she came for was a letter. I literally have no idea how that happened. But I know there was an awkward dance inside me: seeing Aroha, feeling self-conscious at my health altar, knowing Aroha is a target for the health colonisers who know best how she should live her life and who have provided me with a series of medical things I must do to her while she attends my altar.

These things do not include seeing Aroha or laughing with Aroha or hearing Aroha explain that she drives drunk because her post-traumatic anxiety is so severe she would otherwise need to stay home but she prefers to work.

And I wonder if maybe Aroha did that smear because she sensed that dance in me and maybe she felt bad for me with my computer full of grand delusions, or maybe it was because I happen to be in a room with a faulty office chair that sometimes does a sudden descent if I sit down quickly, and so I ended up looking ridiculous with my knees around my chin and that made us both giggle.

Or maybe it wasn't that, maybe she had wanted me to 'smear her mea' all along but just couldn't say until she knew I had heard the bit about the trauma and let it be there between us, as it will always be between the coloniser and the dispossessed: the anguish of many generations, a thing hovering for us to notice, wonder about and handle with care because maybe it is in that hovering thing that the kōrero about health really begins.

I don't know the answer, but I know that this cross-cultural post-colonisation health kōrero is only just beginning. After 30 years as a doctor I am barely getting to understand in some hazy form what is really going on in that room.

It's hard to tell Aroha's story. I don't want to create negative stereotyping that reinforces racist rhetoric about hopeless Māori. Of course there are Pākehā like Aroha and Māori not like Aroha, but I do want us to start in the really hard places, with the stories that make us squirm and despair so much we are compelled to seek collective redemption.

And I'm glad Aroha's smear came back normal.

Whakawhanaungatanga

At medical school these days we teach a lot of cross-cultural communication. We are at the Pākehā end of a country on a journey, and in our earnest academic way we are trying to define concepts like whakawhanaungatanga. I can recall when this word first came into our teaching; it took me a long time to work out how to say it and I always felt such a long word must have a bit of a story, but we were told whakawhanaungatanga meant 'establishing connection'.

In the communication skills laboratory we started teaching students to make connection with Māori patients, played by actors, by asking them about themselves, and some braver students got as far as, 'Where is your home marae?' If there was an exam, they would have got an A for that.

Reflecting on it now, 'communication skills laboratory' seems like an unlikely venue for an authentic cross-cultural connection. I can't imagine what it was like for the actor playing the kuia to walk up the stairs under portraits of Edwardian professors, past signs to toxicology and anatomical dissection and directions to the quality and safety unit. It was a place both grand and dismal.

We had a sense that a Māori doctor might perform some extra mysterious ritual of whakawhanaungatanga — perhaps by connecting their whakapapa with the patients' — but back then medical school was still a Pākehā sort of place, so whakawhanaungatanga got translated into a slightly uncomfortable level of self-disclosure, like telling the patient where you were born or that you had no children.

About that time I was up north for some other reason, and I thought of my old friend Mere.

Lovely Mere, I have not seen you for 30 years.

Mere, who was brought up around whānau in a hau kāinga.

Mere, who used to swing poi with her aunties and cousins for busloads of tourists at the Travelodge.

Mere, who did all the laundry in our flat because she didn't trust I would separate the tea towels from the bath towels. It was a mystery to me why you would.

And I thought so much about Mere she appeared in front of me.

Beautiful Mere, who has had seven children but gave one away to her cousin because it was the right thing to do.

Beautiful Mere, who helps lost youth find their whānau.

Mere, who tells me she is not a fluent te reo speaker and doesn't go so much for te ao Māori because she believes in a Christian god.

'Mere,' I ask, 'what is whakawhanaungatanga?'

'Āe,' she says, smiling, 'it's so great you are teaching this. You're right, it is about establishing connection.'

I made the tea.

'Whakawhanaungatanga,' she says when I return. 'Āe, it's like creating a safe vessel for a big kōrero.'

'Kōrero,' I say, trying to repeat her soft sequence of vowels. 'Sorry, Mere, I am so bad at pronunciation.'

She laughs. 'But I think you get it. Whakawhanaungatanga, it's listening with the body, looking with the heart. It's not just in your mind, Lucy. Your wairua meets their wairua.'

We drink the tea. And I tell Mere about where I was born.

I'm failing as a pro-equity practitioner

I'm trying to be a pro-equity practitioner but I'm not doing so well. Pro-equity means that I strive to give my patients the best possible treatments and therefore the best outcomes for their physical health. But where I work now the ill health is overwhelming. My inbox of letters and results is laden with stories of people who will become health inequity statistics. People here die young. It's heartbreaking.

Today I'm worrying about a young Pasifika woman with type 2 diabetes who has had a glycated haemoglobin over 150 for five years. This level for diabetes is alarming — a glycated haemoglobin over 60 is hazardous. She is 26 years old. I know type 2 diabetes is much more aggressive in the young; in a few years there will be damage to her kidneys, her eyes, her nerves, her blood vessels and her heart. She may have problems in pregnancy.

I did well when I saw her eight months ago. She looked at me respectfully. She even had a first shot of Trulicity and she was so excited about how easy this was going to be, and could she tell her sister about this new wonder drug for diabetes where you only inject once a week? But we have never seen her again. She didn't ever pick up the prescription and she doesn't answer our calls. I have sent texts full of encouragement and lightness and, yes, doses of aroha but still she has not come in the door.

I'm wondering if the door is the problem. It's not her door, it's mine. When I go through that door, I'm entering my place in the world. I am probably carrying my packed lunch of homemade goddess bowl because I'm concerned about my cholesterol even though I'm guessing my life expectancy will be decades longer than the lives of the patients I am seeing. Or the ones I am not seeing.

I'm unsure why she won't come through my door because I'm thinking I'm pretty friendly, but I know that isn't enough. I'm wondering if maybe the door means time and cost and leaving behind fanau obligations, or perhaps it opens up the shame of the scales and maybe an unpaid bill and the blood test not being good enough and the doctor looking disappointed while trying to be nice because the doctor knows a pro-equity practitioner is measured on how well they get the blood sugars and blood pressures down and the life expectancy up. In truth, I'm scared because the stakes are high — young people are dying.

I know that any cross-cultural communication is going to be tricky, and I even get that medicine in itself is a cultural construct. Our health outcomes and health literacy are actually medical outcomes and medical literacy as defined by our world view; we measure health outcomes of the individual, specifically the individual's body. Another view of health may see outcomes differently, perhaps in ways incomprehensible to me, where collective outcomes supersede individual ones. Perhaps spiritual outcomes supersede the body.

But I'm back to worrying about this lovely young woman and the one in her twenties who needs a valve replacement for her rheumatic heart disease, who is so polite when I meet her but never gets to appointments and will probably never get to the operating table. And the man in his thirties already on dialysis who probably won't get a kidney transplant because his second name is D.N.A., Did Not Attend: appointments, GPs, scans, blood tests, specialist clinics.

Did Not Attend is such a common label in the health service, given with such judgement and lack of curiosity, and resulting in such lack of care and consideration from overstretched health care workers who feel frustrated and dismissive of patients who just don't turn up for appointments. As if Did Not Attend is some irreparable breach of contract, although the contract was negotiated on our terms, the breaches defined by us.

What is it that I am not understanding here? I am wondering if D.N.A might be reinterpreted as Door Needs Attention. And I am wondering if someone from that young woman's world needs to help her through? Maybe I should use the Pasifika nursing service more? Bring the fanau in?

But there's still a problem with that door between her life and my room full of medicines and swivel chairs and allocated spaces of time for individual appointments and waiting rooms full of happy health promotion posters. And I am thinking how strange my world must feel to her.

+

And now I am remembering the beautiful things I have experienced working in this community: the care of the collective, multigenerational homes where disabled children and the old people are cared for by family. Like the fanau who cared for their head-injured child for 10 years in a hospital bed in the living room. The father told me, 'We were blessed to have him.'

I am meeting my own Palagi assumptions about the way life should be. Something else is important here. Something bigger than me.

I am remembering someone telling me about the Samoan concept of the vā, the meeting of two worlds, the sacred tapu relational space, where unity takes precedence over individuality. The vā 'connects and holds separate entities and things together in unity'.[1]

I am not even sure what this means in practice and I'm wondering how a Samoan relational space might feel different to a Palagi one? I have my own cultural ways of relating but I sense the need to get up from my swivel chair, leave my beliefs on the desk, take a step towards and allow myself to be folded into a collective story. Politely. And respectfully.

Kaitiakitanga

After a year of immersion in te ao Māori I stood in a wharenui and presented my kaitiakitanga model for 20 minutes without notes or PowerPoint. I couldn't have imagined being able to do that when I started. At the beginning I was fretting about whether Pākehā should even feel entitled to join such a kaupapa.

I had enrolled in Kaitiakitanga — Bicultural Professional Supervision: a mātauranga Māori way of seeing relationships of care and support. There would be eight weekend noho marae over eight months. I was terrified.

Initially I situated myself as 'other' but we were met by a kaiako who told us, 'We will greet the mana in all of you.' Everyone has value. Āki the mana, draw out the mana, see the mana. Mana greets mana.

I heard that in te ao Pākehā we say, 'I think, therefore I am', but in te ao Māori we say, 'I belong, therefore I am'. And I experienced the collective. The collective learns together, eats together, cleans the whare together, washes dishes together, sings together, sleeps together, laughs together, prays together, wonders together, heals together. Our collective mauri, our life force, binds us. The collective does not let us fall behind, suffer alone or feel 'other'. Whiria te tangata, weave the people together.

I learned about being Pākehā, again and again and again, my head banging against the window between me and te ao Māori.

Thinking I could see through but banging against my Pākehā insides, my thinking, my embodiment of self.

I learned that a kupu is not a word because translation between cultures is essentially problematic. Words and kupu have meanings that reflect ways of seeing life and the cosmos, ways of inhabiting time and space, so that aroha is not love and kaitiakitanga is not guardianship but both represent complex ways of being and living. I was trying to understand a way of being Māori that for some is like breathing and realised how much I breathe Pākehā. The hau, the breath, the vital essence that connects us with all other living creatures. Māori hau, Pākehā hau. We share breath.

I learned to STFU and just whakarongo, to listen, to hear, to feel, to smell, to taste, to sense, to perceive. In an oral tradition to listen is to learn. I would think, well, at least I understood whakarongo, then months later realise that rongo is also peace and whaka is to move towards. Whakarongo: listen, with intention towards peace. I learned about noticing our intention: a tangata whai mahara is one who is consciously aware and alert to possibilities and meanings.

+

I learned a new verb: to te aka. *Te Aka* is the Māori dictionary; I te aka-ed my way through the year. A wero is a challenge that upholds mana; a wānanga is a discussion with aroha and māramatanga, a wānanga kaitiaki is therefore a different sort of consultation; aroha is building a bridge to the disconnected — aro, paying attention to, hā, the breath; māramatanga is new understandings, enlightenment, the wairua guides you there. Wairua practice feels better for the soul than self-care — self-care isn't in *Te Aka* because we are whānau, not alone but connected.

Whakawhanaungatanga, the intention to see you as my whānau, as my human kin; whakapapa . . . a series of never-ending beginnings (actually that was Moana Jackson not *Te Aka*[1]), we are just a small blip in the current between the tūpuna and the mokopuna; karakia ignite the connectivity between us, the natural world, the tūpuna, the atua and a wairua realm where there is no time no place no physicality . . . just when I think I am getting it, someone says knowing is not just in the mind; we know in our tinana, our bodies sense it. We know in our wairua, our tūpuna, the tūps, will guide us.

I learned about kaitiakitanga. Akiaki i te tī o te tangata. Draw out the light, seek the light, see the light in the other person. That is kaitiakitanga. Find the light switch and turn it on, do this even in the dark, even if they are hara and even if you are a bit scared or repulsed or riri or raru or wīwī wāwā or pōuri. Keep looking for a switch and if there is no power find the light somewhere. In you or them. Share the light. Āe. Kaitiakitanga.

I have been a manuhiri on the fringes of te ao Māori and I have returned to te ao Pākehā changed. And grateful. My world opened. I came as 'other' and experienced manaakitanga.

Where is all this leading in my life and my work as a GP? You want learning outcomes, 1–10 on Likert scales, boxes ticked?

Maybe I'm waiting for a sign from my tūps and wondering how to let the wairua guide me.

A message to my younger self

- There's a shitload of stuff you need to know that you haven't been taught. So, be curious. Ask questions, don't accept answers. Not much is true or black or white. Be a grey area specialist.
- Listen to your patients because they will teach you about life, and it is life you will swim alongside every day.
- Be a good diagnostician, but don't deliver your diagnoses too proudly.
- Don't be a dick.
- Objectivity is great in an emergency or a medical conundrum, but not many of those happen in general practice, so don't let objectivity block your senses.
- You need sense. And *to* sense.
- Be suspicious of evidence carved into stone tablets. Evidence will change multiple times in your career and sometimes go around in circles to the place it started. Follow it but trust your instinct.
- Be happy not knowing. Sometimes it's not you that needs to know.
- Don't pronounce your opinions too emphatically because you'll be backtracking in a nanosecond.

+ Don't be a tosser.
+ Being a scientist can be fun but be prepared to be a mechanic or magician or cheerleader or a sponge to be squeezed out later.
+ Sense when you have got it wrong. Don't blame the patient. Even a little.
+ Keep off high horses.
+ Sit in with your nurses; they could teach you a thing or two.
+ Sit in the waiting room once in your life, and witness the power of welcome, and the sound of grace down a telephone.
+ It's not all about you.
+ Tick boxes for the bureaucrats then tell them about real life. It's the healing of stories that will fix their statistics.
+ Always guard some place for storing secrets.
+ Realise the patient is interviewing you as much as you them. As well they might.
+ Don't harass the smokers and drinkers; you are asking them to give up their best friends. Ask to meet their friends, yarn with their friends and see where they fit in the story.
+ Don't lecture the vaccine hesitant. Love them like you mean it and tell them to come back when they need another shot of that.
+ Don't pass judgement on the waist circumference, because later when they see themselves naked, they will remember your gaze of righteousness.
+ Don't lecture the non-compliant because their relationship with your pills might be indecipherably messy, in a way that cannot be said to a doctor who insists they must be swallowed.

+ Make your patients' tails wag.
+ Be yourself.
+ Prescribe yourself liberally because you could be the drug; the pill called listening, hope, kindness, reassurance, laughter and love.
+ Hold hope like a life depends on it. It might.
+ Be in terror when the stakes are high but know that it is always too soon to panic. You can cry in the toilets later.
+ Look like you can be tough, but mostly be soft or light or care full, or comfortable teetering on your back foot.
+ Admire your professors but trust your own wisdom.
+ Know your colleagues. I mean *really* know your colleagues: their birthdays, their kids' names, who they pray to, what makes them quiver and hoot. Go towards them when they trip or cry or disappear or become embittered. Even if they are dicks or tossers.
+ And stop trying to be perfect. You're not Jesus.
+ Know yourself. Greet yourself kindly as you walk life's 'good enough' path with the rest of us.
+ Laugh. Laugh at yourself, laugh at medicine, laugh at the craziness of what we are trying to do in so little time.
+ Know that things can be made better, starting with yourself.
+ Know that you are marvellous. When the voices of doubt creep in, when the stuff of life humbles you, when you are drowning in the shame of failure, remember, you are still marvellous.
+ Stop trying to fix things.
+ Fix the things you can.

+ Don't be grandiose. The patient is on the hero's journey, not you.
+ Learn to love, even the unlovable.
+ Eliminate internal eye rolls.
+ Sit steady in the storms that pass through your room, hold on tight, be unrocked.
+ And trust. Because in the end that is the treatment.
+ Be a safe place for stories. You.
+ Be a story doctor. Some stories are short. Others are a complex labyrinth with no end in sight. Some stories will make you rage or cry or keel over with exhaustion but be still and breathe and take the blood pressure if you need to.
+ But know this: the blood pressure, the X-ray, the diagnosis and the prescription are just characters in the story of a life, but they are never the main character.
+ And neither are we.

Glossary

There are many meanings for the words in this list. For this glossary the meanings relate to the context of their use in this book.

āki to encourage, draw out

aroha love, concern, compassion, empathy

ātaahua brave, honest

atua ancestors with continuing influence, god, deity

auē a cry or howl

awa river

fofō Samoan traditional massage or healer

hā breath, essence

hau vital essence, vitality (of a person, place or object), breath

hau kāinga true home

hāngī earth oven; the food cooked in it

hapū pregnant; one's kinship group; whānau sharing descent from a common ancestor

hara in violation of a tapu; to commit a sin or crime; offend, violate, transgress

harakeke New Zealand flax, *Phormium tenax*

hinengaro mind, thought, intellect

iwi katoa wider support systems; health/support services and systems; the collective

kai food; to eat

kaiako teacher

kaiāwhina helper, assistant, contributor, counsel, advocate

kāinga home, village, settlement

kāinga mahinga kai a place for food gathering or cultivation; garden

kaitiakitanga to be a caregiver, custodian; guardianship

karakia prayer, ritual chant

karanga call of welcome to visitors onto a marae

kaumātua elder, a person of status within the whānau

kaupapa philosophy of a person, group or organisation; topic or matter for discussion

kōrero discussion, conversation, narrative, story

koro grandfather

kōwhaiwhai painted scroll patterns, commonly used on meeting house rafters

kuia grandmother, female elder

mahi work

mana prestige, power, status, spiritual power

mana motuhake mana through self-determination and control over one's own destiny

manaaki to support, protect, show respect; generosity and care for others

manaakitanga the process and enaction of manaaki

manuhiri visitor, guest

māramatanga new understandings, enlightenment, insight

matai Samoan chief

mātauranga knowledge, wisdom, understanding

matemate-ā-one profound affection and longing for one's land and home

maunga mountain

mauri life force, vital essence

moko tattoo; mokopuna

moko kauae moko on the chin

mokopuna grandchild, descendent

noa to be free from the extensions of tapu

noho marae overnight stay on a marae

pā Māori village; a hill fort or defensive settlement

pepeha introduction to identify connections to tangata and whenua

pōuri distressed, gloomy, mournful, disheartened, in the dark, not understanding

pōwhiri welcome ceremony onto a marae

raru in difficulty, perplexed, troubled

riri aggressive, enraged, violent

rongo to hear, perceive; peace

taiao natural world, physical environment

tangata whai mahara person seeking to have understanding, be alert to possibilities and meanings

taniwha monster, powerful or formidable creature

taonga treasure, including for social or cultural value

tapu sacred, prohibited, restricted, under atua protection

tauiwi foreigner, European, non-Māori

taulasea Samoan traditional herbal and spiritual healer

Te Kōhanga Reo Māori language preschool

tikanga correct procedure or protocol, customs, values and practices

tinana the body; the real, actual self (as opposed to an apparition)

tino rangatiratanga self-determination, sovereignty, autonomy, self-government

tohunga skilled person, priest or healer chosen by the community for their expertise

tokotoko walking stick

tukutuku symbolic lattice work, often used around the walls of the wharenui

tupuna ancestor

tūpuna ancestors

vā Samoan sacred relational space

waharoa gateway, main entranceway

wahine woman

wāhine women

wairua spirit of a person; soul, essence, atmosphere, feeling

waka huia container for taonga

wānanga to meet and discuss, especially with aroha and māramatanga; Māori educational place

wero challenge that upholds mana

whaka- to move towards

whakamā shame, embarrassment; to be ashamed, shy, embarrassed

whakapapa genealogy, history

whakarongo to listen, hear, perceive, sense, especially with an intention towards peace

whakatere expert navigation skills

whakawhanaungatanga establishing safe connection, relating well to others

whare house, building

wharekai dining hall, place to serve and eat food

wharenui meeting house, main building of a marae where guests stay

whenua land, country, nation

wīwī wāwā to be all over the place, physically or spiritually; a bit lost

Notes

Pākehā doctor, Māori patient

1 Michael Field, *Mau: Samoa's struggle for freedom* (Polynesian Press, 1984).
2 Wiremu NiaNia, Allister Bush and David Epston, *Collaborative and Indigenous Mental Health Therapy: Tātaihono — Stories of Māori healing and psychiatry* (Routledge, 2017), 144–47.
3 Mason Durie, 'A Maori Perspective of Health', *Social Science and Medicine* 20, no. 5 (1982): 483–86, https://doi.org/10.1016/0277-9536(85)90363-6.
4 Suzanne Pitama, Tania Huria and Cameron Lacey, 'Improving Māori health through Clinical Assessment: Waikare o te Waka o Meihana', *New Zealand Medical Journal* 127, no. 1393 (2014): 107–19.

We can do better

1 Emma Espiner, *Getting Better: A year in the life of a Māori medical student*, podcast, Radio New Zealand, https://www.rnz.co.nz/programmes/getting-better

Narrating our selves

1 Megan Cook, 'Women's Movement: Health, Fertility and Education', *Te Ara — the Encyclopedia of New Zealand*, 5 May 2011, www.TeAra.govt.nz/en/ephemera/27921/girls-can-do-anything
2 Martha Morseth, 'Would You Trust This Woman with Your Life?', *More*, 1983, 28–37.
3 Hunter K. Montgomery, *Doctors' Stories: The Narrative Structure of Medical Knowledge* (Princeton University Press, 1991).
4 Ian R. McWhinney, *A Textbook of Family Medicine* (Oxford University Press, 1989).
5 Ibid.
6 Eric J. Cassell, 'The Nature of Suffering and the Goals of Medicine', *New England Journal of Medicine* 306, no. 11 (1982): 639–45 (639).

7 Iona Heath, '"Uncertain clarity": Contradiction, meaning and hope', *British Journal of General Practice* 49, no. 445 (1999): 651–57.

8 Donald Schön, *Educating the Reflective Practitioner: Toward a new design for teaching and learning in the professions* (Jossey-Bass, 1987), 26.

9 Matthew Gothill and David Armstrong, 'Dr No-body: The Construction of the doctor as an embodied subject in British general practice 1955–97', *Sociology of Health and Illness* 21, no. 1 (1999): 1–12.

Sleeping with the ancestors

1 Moana Jackson, 'Where to Next? Decolonisation and the Stories of the Land', in *Imagining Decolonisation*, ed. Rebecca Kiddle (Bridget Williams Books, 2020), 154.

The Zen of general practice

1 '2018 Workforce Survey', The Royal New Zealand College of General Practitioners, https://www.rnzcgp.org.nz/RNZCGP/News/College_news/2019/2018_Workforce_Survey_Results.aspx; 10 per cent scored themselves at 0 or 'not at all burnt out' (personal communication).

Story doctor

1 Arthur Franks, *The Wounded Storyteller: Body, illness and ethics* (University of Chicago Press, 1995).

2 Kathy Weingarten, 'Witnessing, Wonder and Hope', *Family Process* 39, no. 4 (2000): 393.

3 Ian R. McWhinney, *A Textbook of Family Medicine* (Oxford University Press, 1989), 84–85.

4 Gillie Bolton, *Reflective Practice: Writing and professional development* (Sage, 2014).

I'm failing as a pro-equity practitioner

1 Jemaima Tiatia, 'Commentary on "Cultural Diversity Across the Pacific": Samoan cultural constructs of emotion, New Zealand-born Samoan youth suicidal behaviours, and culturally competent human services', *Journal of Pacific Rim Psychology* 6, no. 2 (2012): 75–79, https://doi 10.1017/prp.2012.9

Kaitiakitanga

1 Moana Jackson, 'Where to Next? Decolonisation and the Stories of the Land', in *Imagining Decolonisation*, ed. Rebecca Kiddle (Bridget Williams Books, 2020), 139.

Author's note

Inevitably a book about the experience of being a doctor has to include stories about patients, but writing about real patients is incredibly problematic. The stories told in consultation rooms must remain confidential.

The commonly used practice of changing identifying data such as name, gender and diagnosis is also problematic in small towns in a small country, where people can be recognised. So these are composite stories, drawing on multiple memories and experiences, to build whole new stories.

Other writers tell me that readers who know an author always think the characters in the book are based on them. I think this will inevitably happen but I would not want people to be distressed by this. All I can say is that none of the stories bear more than a fragment of any story from any patient I have known. If a fragment feels like a fragment of you, please know that the story I have written is not now about you: it is about me.

He whakamihi

Thank you to my mum, who loved words and knew the power of them, to my dad, who before anyone else showed me how to be a doctor, and taught me to question with rigorous enthusiasm, and to my brother Sean, who first introduced me to the long meandering sentence. You would all have loved this book.

To my whānau, who have taught me much about life, who take the piss, keep me in my place and make me hold my end up, all with a good giggle and a lot of love.

To Barbara Fountain, editor at *New Zealand Doctor Rata Aotearoa*, for inviting me to write a monthly column on anything I liked, which was an absolute gift. *Everything but the Medicine* started there.

Versions of some of these chapters first appeared in *New Zealand Doctor*, *Corpus* and the *Journal of Primary Health Care*. I am grateful to their editors for permission to publish them here in adapted form.

To Nicola Legat from Massey University Press for her steady hand, enthusiasm and guidance. To project editor Anna Jackson-Scott for being there to explain the process. And to copy editor Tracey Lowndes for being beautifully pedantic and spotting every clumsy sentence. To designer Kate Barraclough for transforming a Word document into a beautiful book.

To Charlotte Yates for patiently recording this tale.

To Glenn Colquhoun for making me print out those stories, lay them on the floor, get them in the right order, then take them to Warehouse Stationery to bind them up and send them to him. Such kindness and belief.

To my niece Ruby Porter for encouraging poetry. To Anthony Doesburg for showing me how a lazy sentence can be cut, kinked and reassembled without losing any of the nuance. To my manuscript assessors, Sue Reidy, Geoff Walker, Caroline Barron and Alie Benge. I would never have got there without you.

To Pat Farry, Hamish Wilson, Chrys Jaye and the team who dreamed up and taught the Master of General Practice programme at Otago Medical School. Thank you for helping me understand medicine through the lens of social science. To the tutors and students at the Center for Narrative Practice for helping me understand how stories work, including our own. To my kaitiakitanga whānau, thanks for making wairua real and manaakitanga a way of being.

To Simon, the loveliest and craziest of dads, who could always put medicine, magic and laughter in the same room. To my son Johnny for being proud of his mum and whose enthusiastic track changes were thought-provoking and perceptive. To my son Fergus, who usually says, 'Haha. I love it, Mum.'

To my partner, Lizzi, who has taught me more about kindness than anyone and who has read these stories multiple times and never seems to get bored — for all those conversations, love, laughter and belief. And for creating a beautiful image for the book cover.

To Katerina, our daughter, for being a beautiful part of the story.

To the colleagues who have listened, understood, laughed, cried and wondered with me. And finally, and mostly, to the patients I have met and the stories they have shared. Thank you.

About the author

Lucy O'Hagan entered Otago Medical School in the first class to be half female and graduated in the year of the Cartwright Inquiry. She has studied the sociology, anthropology and philosophy of medicine, as well as narrative practice.

She has been a rata hauora/general practitioner for over 30 years and has worked in a huge range of contexts: rural tourist town, shearing gang clinics, urban iwi-run services and free clinics for the homeless. She currently works at Oratoa Cannons Creek in East Porirua in a predominantly Māori Pasifika practice owned by Ngāti Toa Rangatira.

Lucy has been mentoring GP trainees for over 20 years, including teaching consultation skills and reflective practice. She is a well-known GP writer, speaker and performer who has written plays, given addresses and performances at conferences and written a monthly column for *New Zealand Doctor Rata Aotearoa* since 2017.

In 2024 she recorded stories and reflections she had written during the pandemic. *Waiting for Covid* is available on podcast platforms.

MASSEY UNIVERSITY PRESS

First published in 2025 by Massey University Press
Private Bag 102904, North Shore Mail Centre
Auckland 0745, New Zealand
www.masseypress.ac.nz

Design by Kate Barraclough
Cover artwork by Lizzi Yates: *Still life in scraps*, 2023

A catalogue record for this book is available from the National Library of New Zealand

Printed and bound in China by Everbest Investment Ltd

ISBN: 978-1-991309-07-5
eISBN: 978-1-991309-08-2
aISBN: 978-1-991309-20-4